Saving Lives, Minimally Invasive: Cell Therapy for Abdominal Aortic Aneurysms

Monty

CHAPTER I

INTRODUCTION

Abdominal aortic aneurysms (AAAs) are localized expansions of the abdominal aorta (infrarenal part of the largest artery supplying blood to the body). They are a multifactorially determined conditions triggered by genetic predispositions and/or environmental factors [1]. Although the disease etiology remains largely unknown, infiltration of inflammatory cells, smooth muscle cell (SMC) apoptosis, breakdown of elastic matrix (a key structural extracellular matrix component), abnormal accumulation of collagen and oxidative stress are among manifested indications of AAAs pathology [2]. Chronic persistence of the inflammatory process aggravates enzymatic breakdown of the elastic matrix by inflammatory cells resulting in loss of stretch and recoil properties, and subsequent exuberant but transient deposition of collagen by aneurysmal smooth muscle cells that causes transient stiffening of the aorta wall prior to weakening and fatal flow stress-induced rupture [1], [2].

The major challenge in therapeutic reversal of AAAs as in other proteolytic disorders involving elastic tissues/organs (e.g., chronic obstructive pulmonary disease or COPD, pelvic organ prolapse or POP etc.) is the degeneration of the elastic matrix which is a naturally irreversible process. This is attributed to the poor ability of adult and even more so, diseased cells to synthesize elastin the primary protein component of elastic fibers, beyond the late fetal and early neonatal stages of life, and their inability to replicate the biocomplexity of developmental elastic fiber assembly [3]. Therefore, reversing AAA pathophysiology to a healthy tissue state demands an external stimulus to stimulate elastogenesis and concurrently attenuate chronic proteolysis by overexpressed degradative enzymes called matrix metalloproteases (MMPs).

1.1   Overall goal of the project

Regenerative repair of elastic matrix in the AAA wall is naturally poor due to intrinsically poor elastogenicity of adult and diseased vascular SMCs [4]. In this scenario, cell therapy involving delivery of an alternate, possibly autologous cell type that would exhibit the high contractility of terminally differentiated SMCs in healthy vessels and yet exhibit the high elastogenic potential of SMC progenitor cells in early development would proffer an attractive prospect to stimulate elastogenesis lasting new elastic matrix assembly by diseased SMCs in the AAA wall . Based on prior studies in our lab that demonstrated superior elastogenicity of bone marrow mesenchymal stem cell (BM-MSC)-derived SMCs (BM-SMCs) and their ability to provide pro-elastogenic and anti-proteolytic stimuli to aneurysmal SMCs [5], [6], the overall goal of this study is to understand the pro-elastogenic and anti-proteolytic behavior of BM-MSCs derived SMCs in long term *in vitro* 2D and 3D culture, investigate their fate an *in vivo* rat model of induced AAA, and to seek preliminary evidence of their therapeutic efficacy for AAA treatment.

1.2   Significance and innovation of proposed study

The prevalence of AAA is 3.9% to 7.2% in men and 1.0% to 1.3% in women above 50 years of age and mortality due to ruptured AAAs is 75% to 90% making it the 10th leading cause of death in the US [7]. AAAs are asymptomatic and can rupture without warning. Current management of AAAs involve periodic non-invasive imaging using ultrasonography or MRI to monitor their growth until they reach a critical size deemed to have high rupture risk (~5.5 cm in diameter) at which time surgical intervention is deemed appropriate [8]. Most common surgical interventions are open surgical repair or endovascular repair (EVAR) [9]. Both surgical procedures are highly invasive accompanied by high procedural risks and significant post-surgical complications. This justifies the dire need of alternative minimally invasive treatments to arrest or regress small AAAs during their years-long growth to the critical size. The regenerative therapy addressed by this study based on the use of adult stem cells is thus highly significant especially since even drugs currently in the development pipeline, discussed further in Chapter 2, have been shown to at best provide only anti-proteolytic benefit. I envision my proposed therapy to involve simple intravenous infusion of a cell bolus or single or multiple event, catheter-based infusion of cells into a transiently flow-occluded AAA vessel segment. Upon *in vivo* delivery, it is expected that at a fraction of these cells will home in and engraft in the AAA wall and provide a new source of elastic matrix besides sustained paracrine matrix regenerative and anti-proteolytic cues to stimulate elastic matrix neo-assembly by resident aneurysmal SMCs for long term therapeutic benefit. Since these methods are procedurally simple and are at most minimally invasive, mortality and complications associated with surgery on older, vulnerable patients can be potentially eliminated. Due to their multifunctional benefits, cell therapy with BM-SMCs can potentially provide a significant advantage over current drug-based treatments that show some promise, namely treatment with the MMP inhibitor drug, doxycycline (DOX). While oral DOX therapy has shown some promise in small and larger animal models [refs] in inhibiting MMPs in the AAA wall to slow AAA growth, outcomes in clinical trials has been inconsistent [1], [10]. Moreover, studies have shown that the high clinical doses of DOX adversely inhibits crosslinking of even the limited new elastin produced within the AAA wall, thus eliminating any prospects to arrest or reverse AAA growth. Besides circumventing this issue, BM-SMC therapy could also possibly improve endovascular stent graft detachment from the AAA wall, a frequently encountered problem, by limiting continued expansion of the adjacent AAA wall. Similarly, if the trophic factors contained in the BM-SMC secretome that are necessary and sufficient for their pro-elastogenic/anti-MMP effects are identified, new approaches based on delivery of these agents alone or in combination may be possible, without need to obtain, process, expand, and deliver cells. While use of allogeneic BM-MSCs for cell therapy is acceptable even in the clinic, we expect our study of these cells to guide future investigation of patient derived cells which can potentially enable patient customized treatments.

Based on the information outlined above, the novelty of our research at this point lies in the approach of delivering healthy allogeneic BM-MSC derived BM-SMCs that retain high elastogenic capacity unlike most adult cell types. While SMCs are known to exhibit a continuum of phenotypes ranging between theoretical extremes of synthetic and contractile phenotypes, this study is novel in identifying specific phenotypic coordinates of derived BM-SMCs that are conducive to the cells providing pro-elastogenic, anti-proteolytic, and anti-apoptotic stimuli to aneurysmal SMCs via their paracrine secretions while maintaining high contractility of vascular SMCs. While undifferentiated BM-MSCs are known to home into site of tissue injury to effect repair, the retention of these homing properties by non-terminally differentiated, derived BM-SMCs is largely unknown, on which this study is expected to provide new insight. Innovation in this work also concerns the study of variety of co-culture systems in a collagenous, 3D milieu that can more closely evoke the cellular milieu within elastin-compromised aneurysmal site, and thus likely elicit more closely physiologic responses to provided stimuli. Therefore, the procedural simplicity of our delivery approach combined with the innovation and potential benefits of a regenerative cell therapy will be promising to delay or eliminate need for surgical interventions in the primarily older AAA patients, and thus much reduced associated mortality and complications. Our regenerative cell therapy is thus highly significant because it fulfills a critical clinical need, is innovative, translational and mechanistic.

1.3   General hypothesis

We hypothesize that BM-SMCs demonstrate the ability to home-in and be retained in the AAA site to impart superior pro-elastogenic and anti-proteolytic effect compared to the undifferentiated BM-MSCs.

1.4   Specific aims (SAs)

SA 1. To investigate the long-term retention of the phenotype and elastin regenerative benefits of BM-SMCs in 2D culture.

Synopsis: Cell therapy demands large cell inoculates which requires extensive propagation of BM-SMCs in culture prior to its delivery. Thus, it is implicit that these cells should maintain their differentiated phenotype and superior elastin regenerative and homeostasis properties in long-term 2D culture. For this purpose, we sought to differentiate rat BM-MSCs into BM-SMCs per prior optimized protocol on a fibronectin substrate with transforming growth factor-β (TGF-β) and platelet derived growth factor (PDGF-BB) supplements. The differentiated cells were then propagated under the differentiation condition and also as regular SMCs in an uncoated plastic without supplemental growth factors. The two sets of cells were comparatively assessed for retention of differentiated SMC phenotypic characteristics and their superior elastin regenerative properties (higher elastin synthesis and crosslinking, improved fiber formation, lower MMP expression versus control cells, healthy rat aortic SMCs (RASMCs) and undifferentiated BM-MSCs.

SA 2. To investigate in culture the modulatory effects of a 3D collagenous tissue milieu on *de novo* elastin synthesis by BM-SMCs and their paracrine pro-matrix regenerative effects on aneurysmal SMCs (EaRASMCs).

Synopsis: Cells delivered to the AAA wall encounter a collagenous tissue microenvironment. To evoke this, BM-SMCs differentiated and propagated under conditions deemed favorable in SA 1, were statically cultured as standalone as well as in co-culture with aneurysmal SMCs (EaRASMCs) within compacted collagen gels and assessed for quantitative and qualitative (elastic matrix crosslinking, fiber formation and size, stability against proteolysis etc.).

SA 3. To investigate the ability of BM-SMCs to home into the AAA wall, their bio-distribution and retention post-delivery and to provide the initial evidence of their pro-elastogenic and anti-proteolytic benefits.

Synopsis: Effective cell therapies rely on the methods of cell delivery, bio-distribution post-delivery and ability of the cells to home and retain in the target site to impart the desired benefits. For this purpose, in experiment 1, the expression of receptor involved in homing (mainly CXCR4) was assessed *in vitro*. Experiment 2 was focused on delivering the cells. For this, the bolus of 2×10^6 cells were injected via tail vein injection in the aneurysm induced rat. The cells were tracked using IVIS spectrum CT and at end point the aortae were harvested for histology and biochemical assays to observe the benefits of cell therapy.

1.5 Organization of book

Chapter II will provide a comprehensive literature review on histological and anatomical features of abdominal aorta, progression of AAA, elastin protein synthesis, fiber formation and homeostasis, challenges in elastin regeneration and current management of AAAs including the state of art in elastic tissue repair. Pertinent to the last-mentioned topic, the chapter will also discuss different regenerative approaches, pros and cons of each of those, stem cells as an alternative approach for regenerative repair of AAAs and pros and cons of the same.

Chapter III will describe the long-term retention of phenotype and superior elastogenicity of mesenchymal stem cells derived smooth muscle cells in 2D culture.

Chapter IV will shed light on behavior of these derived cells in a 3D collagenous culture which is evocative of de-elasticized AAA tissue milieu.

Chapter V details the *in vivo* cell delivery study, bio-distribution of cells, the evidence of their pro-elastogenic and anti-proteolytic effects at tissue level.

Chapter VI will address the limitations of the study, future directions and overall conclusion.

CHAPTER II

BACKGROUND

2.1   Overview of Extracellular Matrix (ECM)

The extracellular matrix (ECM) is a dynamic, intricate and complex 3D structure surrounding the cells in all tissues. It provides an (a) essential physical scaffolding for the cellular components of tissues and (b) biochemical and biomechanical cues that are critical for tissue morphogenesis, differentiation and homeostasis [11]. The ECM also modulates the most fundamental characteristics of cells such as proliferation, adhesion, migration, polarity, differentiation and apoptosis. These cellular functions are initiated by binding of cells to the ECM through ECM receptors (e.g., integrins, discoidin domain receptors, syndecans) [11]. It also serves as reservoir for various growth factors and signaling molecules that serve to elicit signal transduction and regulation gene transcription and hence direct the morphology and physiological function of cells [12].

2.2　Major ECM components

The ECM primarily consists of non-fibrillar components such as water, proteins and polysaccharide and fibrillar components such as collagens, fibronectin, laminin and elastin. However, the physical, topological and biochemical composition of the ECM is highly heterogenous and tissue specific [12]. The mechanical and biochemical characteristics of individual organs (e.g., tensile and compressive strength, elasticity, extracellular homeostasis and water retention) are influenced by the tissue-specific composition and structural organization of their ECM [12].

2.2.1　Collagen

Collagen is one of the major structural components of ECM. It provides tensile strength to the tissue, regulate cell adhesion, helps in chemotaxis and migration as well as direct tissue development [13]. Collagens are typically transcribed and secreted by fibroblasts as procollagen and undergoes several post translational modifications and lysyl oxidase mediated crosslinking forming the triple helical collagen superstructures as shown in **Figure 1** [13]. Approximately28 different types of collagens are found in ECM and collagen molecules are formed by 3 polypeptide strands called α-chains [13]. Each α-chain assumes left-handed helix and these 3 helices are twisted together creating homo- or heterotrimeric triple helices. α-chains are composed of repeating sequence of three amino acids Gly-X-Y patterned as Gly-Pro-X or Gly-X-Hyp where X can be any other amino acid residues. Some covalent crosslinkings are present within the helix and between different helices to form collagen fibrils. Fibrils are aggregates of several subunits called tropocollagen and bundles of these fibrils are collagen fibers which helps in resisting shear and tensile force like the high pressure imparted by blood flow to the aorta wall.

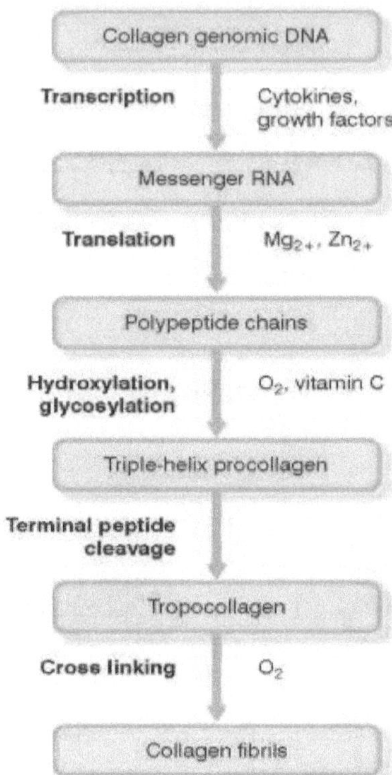

Figure 1: Flowchart showing the process of mature collagen fibril formation

The aorta primarily contains type I and type III collagen, which together account for 80-90% of the total collagen content on a dry weight basis [14]. Other collagen contained in the aorta wall include types IV, V, VI and VIII. The amount and localization of different collagen types however varies according to the region of aorta [15]. For example, the intimal, medial and adventitial layers of healthy aortae contain types I and type III collagen whereas types IV and V are primarily localized in the endothelial and smooth muscle basement membranes [15]. Studies have also shown the localization of types I, III and IV in the intimal and medial layers of the ascending aorta, and distribution of types I and IV throughout the intima and media in the descending thoracic region [14]. Differently, types I and IV are seen in the intimal and medial layers and type III in the adventitial layer of the abdominal aorta [15]. The amount and ratios of different collagen types vary with age, levels of sex hormones, pathologies, etc. For e.g., the stiffening of the aorta wall occurs with ageing likely due to an increment in type-I collagen content [15].

2.2.2   Elastin

Elastin is the primary protein component of elastic fibers, structural ECM components that impart stretch and recoil properties (elasticity) to the tissues subjected to repeated stretch (e.g., blood vessels and lungs) [4]. Unlike collagen which provides strength and flexibility, elastin serves to bring the tissue back to the original shape after stretch and hence helps to maintain tissue integrity. The elastic matrix is described detail in **section 2** below.

2.2.3   Laminin and Fibronectin

Laminin is one of the important components of ECM that intend to self-assemble to create a large network in the basement membrane. It comprises of about 20 glycoproteins assembled into a cross-linked web interwoven with the type IV collagen network via bridging molecules like perlecan. It consists of heterotrimer with one each of α-, β- and γ- chains [16]. Laminins have important role in early embryonic development and organogenesis [16]. They also regulate the differentiation, adhesion, and migration of epithelial cells interacting through multiple cell surface receptors including integrins and cell surface proteoglycans (PGs) [17].

Fibronectin (FN) is a component of the interstitial ECM. It also mediates cell attachment and function [16]. It is a fibril-forming glycoprotein which is structurally a dimer of two identical proteins of 250 kDa covalently attached via disulfide bonds at their C termini. It is ubiquitously expressed in tissues. Different functional motifs on its structure helps fibronectin to interact with GAGs, collagens, fibrin and integrins facilitating matrix organization and cell–matrix interactions [18]. For example, fibronectin serves as a template for proper collagen fibrillogenesis by forming a fibril network engaged by cell surface integrins [16]. Cellular traction force causes FN to be stretched several times over its resting length [18]. As a result of such stretching, cryptic integrin-binding sites within the FN molecule is exposed resulting in pleiotropic changes in cellular behavior [18]. Hence FN acts as an extracellular mechano-regulator in addition to its role in cell migration during development. Studies have also shown the implication of FN in cardiovascular diseases and tumor metastasis [18].

2.2.4   Proteoglycans and Glycosaminoglycans (GAGs)

Proteoglycans (PGs) are macromolecules in the ECM that function as shock absorbers [16]. A classic example is the ECM of cartilage. In dense connective tissues like bone and tendons, contribution of PGs to the properties of the ECM are shadowed by the abundant presence of collagen [19]. Unlike collagen, PGs function to resist compression and serve as space fillers. PGs consist of a core of protein linked to a special class of complex negatively charged polysaccharides called glycosaminoglycans or GAGs [20]. GAGs are linear, anionic, unbranched polysaccharides made up of repeating disaccharide units [20]. GAGs are divided into two groups: sulfated (chondroitin sulfate, heparan sulfate and keratan sulfate) and non-sulfated (hyaluronic acid) GAGs. Often, GAG chains are attached to a single protein core and may link at one end to another GAG resulting in huge macromolecule which may resemble a bottlebrush structure with molecular weights exceeding millions of Daltons [20]. GAGs are extremely hydrophilic and assumes highly extended conformations occupying a huge volume relative to their mass. They have tendency of forming gels even at very low concentration. The negative charges of GAGs attract osmotically active cations like Na^+ which results in suction of large amount of water into the matrix resulting in swelling pressure [19]. In collagen rich matrix containing large quantities of GAGs entrapped in collagen meshes, the swelling pressure is balanced by the tension in the collagen fibers interwoven with the PGs. This swelling pressure and the tension are huge and thus this character makes matrix tough, resilient and resistant to compression like that in cartilage [19].

PGs are extremely diverse in size, shape and chemistry. The classification of PGs is based on their core proteins, localization and GAG composition. They are broadly divided into three main families: small leucine-rich proteoglycans (SLRPs), modular proteoglycans and cell-surface proteoglycans [19], [20]. The functions of each of these has been shown in **Table I** below. Like GAGs, PGs are also highly hydrophilic that readily forms hydrogel enabling matrices that are formed by these molecules to withstand high compressive forces [19]. They perform many sophisticated functions such as to (a) form gels of varying pore sizes and charge densities, which regulate the passage of molecules through the ECM, (b) provide hydrated space around the cells, (c) bind cell signaling molecules like secreted growth factors and other proteins, (d) block, encourage or guide cell migration through the matrix and (e) provide lubrication function and shock absorbing functions [19]. Mutation in PGs genes have also been implicated in many genetic diseases [12], [21]·[22]·[23].

Table I: List of proteoglycans and their respective functions

Family	Example	Function	References
Single Leucine Rich Proteoglycans (SLRPs)	Biglycan, fibromodulin, epiphycan, chondroadherin, podocin, etc.	Activation of signaling pathways like epidermal growth factor receptor (EGFR), regulation of inflammatory response reaction, binding to and activation of TGF β.	[20],[22],[23]
Modular PGs	Perlecan, versican, agrin, collagen type XVIII, etc.	Modulate cell adhesion, migration and proliferation as well as pro- and anti- angiogenic effects.	[20],[23]
Cell-surface PGs	Syndecans and Glypicans	Act as co-receptor to facilitate ligand binding with signaling receptors.	[20]

2.2.5 Cellular receptors and ECM remodeling enzymes

Communication between ECM molecules and cells occurs through the mediation of integrins, syndecans, and other receptors [16]. Integrins are heterodimeric receptors composed of α and β subunits [23]. The integrin family consists of 18 α and 8 β subunits that can assemble into 24 different integrins. Both α and β subunits are transmembrane proteins with large modular extracellular domains, single transmembrane helices, and short cytoplasmic regions that mediate cytoskeletal interactions. Major matrix-binding integrins are the $\beta 1$ integrins which has affinity to fibronectin, collagens, and laminins [16].

Activation of integrins by matrix ligands leads to conformational changes in the integrins which exposes their cytoplasmic domains facilitating binding of focal complex proteins such as the focal adhesion kinase (FAK) and integrin–linked kinase (ILK) [23]. Integrins cluster in the membrane and intracellular proteins including vinculin and talin along with actin stress fibers are assembled into focal adhesion complexes. The integrins subsequently trigger phosphorylation cascades and initiate signaling events including Rho and MAP kinase pathways to affect cell proliferation, differentiation, polarity, contractility, and gene expression in "outside-in" signaling process [16]. Intracellular signals from proteins such as FAK, ILK and talin can conversely induce changes in integrin conformation and activation altering its ligand binding activity in the "inside-out" signaling fashion. Therefore, integrins act as a bi-directional conduit, transmitting signals and providing connections between intra- and extra-cellular compartments [24], [25].

2.3   Major Functions of the ECM

2.3.1   Reservoir

The ECM functions as a structure to sequester growth factors and cytokines. It establishes concentration gradients and regulates spatial and temporal bioavailability of those factors [16]. Specifically, the fibroblast growth factor family strongly binds to heparan sulfate chains of proteoglycans such as perlecan [16]. Heparan sulfate proteoglycans also binds, transports, and activates developmental control factors like Wnt and hedgehog factors. The ECM also stores bioactive fragments released upon limited proteolysis [26]. These fragments regulate physiological and pathological processes including angiogenesis. TGF-β, secreted in latent form, is stored in the ECM and remains inactive until activated by MMP-dependent proteolysis. The ECM also participates in ligand maturation [26].

2.3.2   Chemical and Physical cues

The biochemical properties of the ECM acts as sensors allowing cells to sense and interact with their extracellular environment via various signal transduction pathways [16]. ECM components especially the adhesive proteins like fibronectin, integrin and non-integrin receptors as well as growth factors and associated signaling molecules provide the chemical cues [16]. Distinct cellular responses are triggered by specific sets of receptors interacting with different matrices [16], [24]. The ECM also functions as a physical barrier, an anchorage site, or a movement track for cell migration [26]. The physical properties of the ECM like its rigidity, density, porosity, insolubility and topography (spatial arrangement and orientation) provide physical cues to the cells [26]. Differently, the mechanical properties are mostly sensed by integrins [23]. Matrix stiffness induces integrin clustering, robust focal adhesions and Rho and MAP kinase activation leading to increased proliferation and contractility [23]. Matrix rigidity also regulates cell differentiation. For instance, mesenchymal stem cells favor differentiation towards a neuronal lineage on soft matrices and towards osteogenic lineage on stiff surface [16].

2.4   Elastin and elastic fibers

Elastin is a highly durable and insoluble biopolymer with very limited turnover and estimated half-life of about 70 years in healthy tissues [4]. The monomeric unit of this biopolymer is called tropoelastin which is soluble precursor of elastin. 60 to 70 kDa protein tropoelastin undergoes lysine mediated crosslinking initiated through the action of lysyl oxidase (LOX) to form insoluble elastin. Elastin contributes approximately 90% of constituents of elastic fibers forming the core. Elastic fibers are major components of extracellular matrix which imparts structural integrity to the tissues and acts as dynamic modulator of different biological processes. Elastic fibers provide stretch and recoil properties to all the elastic tissues of vertebrates which helps in maintaining long term functionality of tissues. Elastic fibers are present in all the major organs like arteries, lungs, skin, ligament, vocal cords and elastic cartilage.

2.4.1 Elastin synthesis and fiber assembly

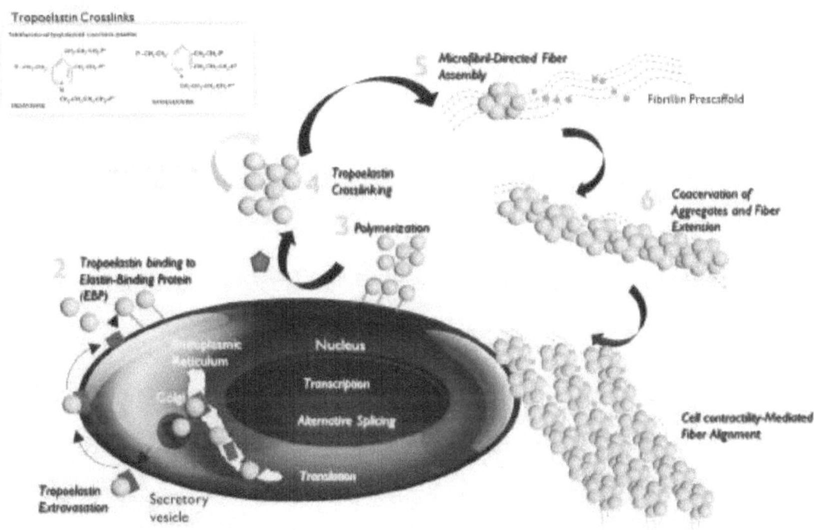

Figure 2: Schematic showing the complex process of elastic fiber formation

Elastin protein synthesis and elastic fiber assembly are highly complex and hierarchical processes as illustrated in the **Figure 2** above. Understanding this complex process is important in order to identify limitations in natural repair and regeneration of elastic matrices and to develop methods to overcome the same. Elastic matrix assembly primarily initiates during the developmental stage and continues until adolescence. Several glycoproteins are involved in this complex process which are regulated at multiple levels.

The first step of the fiber assembly process is secretion of the elastin precursor, tropoelastin. In humans, tropoelastin is encoded by a single copy of gene called *ELN* [27]. *ELN* is synthesized and secreted by smooth muscle cells (SMCs) [27], fibroblasts, endothelial cells, chondroblasts and mesothelial cells during development [28]. The tropoelastin amino acid sequence is well characterized and includes an alternating hydrophobic and hydrophilic domain structure [29]. The hydrophobic domain of the protein consists of repetitive sequences of non-polar amino acids valine, glycine, valine, alanine, proline and glycine (VGVAPG), which account for 82% of the primary sequence [30]. The hydrophilic domain or the crosslinking domain on the other hand is rich in lysine and alanine [3]. Following extensive splicing, matured tropoelastin mRNA is exported from the nucleus and undergoes translation on the surface of rough endoplasmic reticulum(rER) forming a 70 kDa polypeptide [31]. As the polypeptide enters the lumen of rER, it is cleaved and released as single peptide which is transported to the Golgi [32]. Tropoelastin is then exported to the extracellular space by transcytosis which then binds to a chaperone protein called elastin binding protein (EBP) [33]. The EBP binds predominantly to the hydrophobic domains on elastin [33]. Intracellularly, EBP prevents the self-aggregation and degradation of tropoelastin whereas extracellularly, it helps to deliver tropoelastin to the microfibrillar site of fiber formation [32]. Binding of EBP to the microfibrillar galactose-sugars results in the release of tropoelastin from EBP [34]. The EBP is then recycled back to the intracellular space to bind the newly formed tropoelastin molecules [32]. The tropoelastin is released from EBP coacervates. Coacervation is the inverse temperature transition involving extracellular interaction between hydrophobic domains of tropoelastin causing aggregation of molecules with increased temperature [33]. Coacervated molecules are then crosslinked through the action of a copper dependent enzyme called LOX [35]–[37]. LOX catalyzes the oxidative deamination of amino groups on the lysine residues within tropoelastin to form allysine which is the reactive precursor of variety of inter and intramolecular crosslinks found in elastin [37]. Condensation of two allysine residues on one tropoelastin and one allysine residue and one lysine residue in another molecule results in formation of desmosine crosslinks [38] **(Figure 3)**. The crosslinked tropoelastin molecule is deposited on the microfibrillar pre-scaffold [39]. The pre-scaffold (a) provides spatial co-ordination and alignment to coalescing tropoelastin nuclei towards their extension and crosslinking to form mature elastic fibers, (b) maintain fiber integrity, and (c) facilitate biomechanical transduction of adjacent cells by elastic fibers [39]. The mature elastic fiber formed exhibits a cross-sectional diameter of about 300 nm to 2 um with a central core of alkali-insoluble crosslinked elastin surrounded by microfibrils [39]. The microfibrils also act as a scaffold maintaining the structural integrity of elastic fibers as well as serve as a reservoir to various growth factors (GFs) [39].

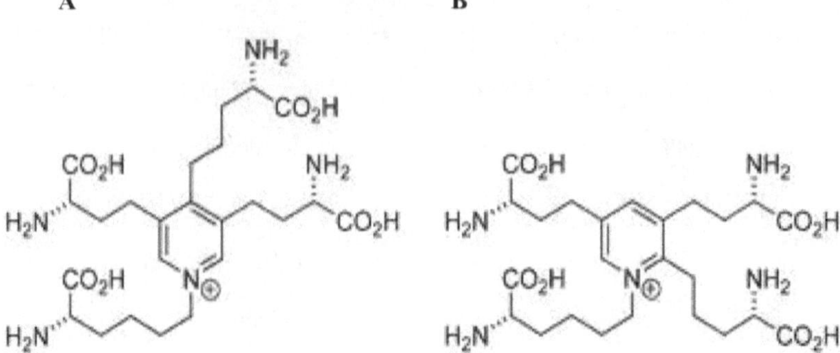

Figure 3: Structure of (A) Desmosine and (B) Isodesmosine

2.4.2 Structure, function and properties

As mentioned earlier, the primary structure of tropoelastin comprises of alternating hydrophobic (containing highly conserved VGVAPG amino acid sequence) and crosslinking domains (rich in lysine and alanine residues) [40], [41]. The secondary protein structure consists of alternating α-helices (crosslinking domains) and β-sheets (hydrophobic domains) encoded by separate exons as shown in the **Figure 4** below [42].

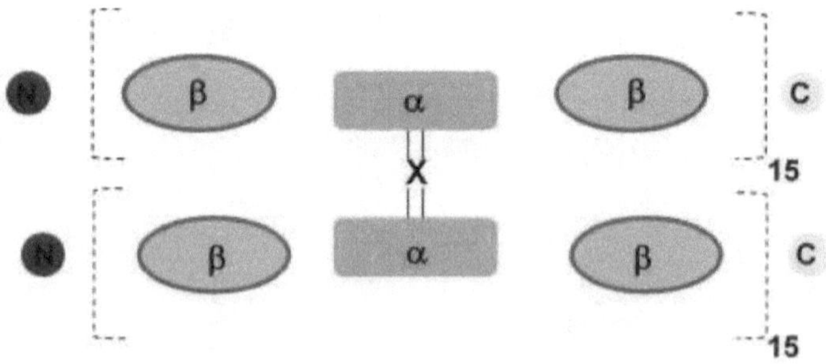

Figure 4: Secondary structure of elastin showing alternating α-helix and β-sheets

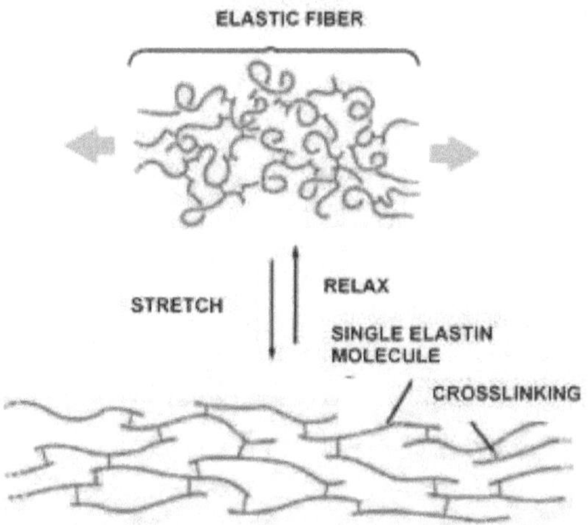

Figure 5: Elastin stretch and recoil showing crosslinks limiting the extent of stretch

The crosslinking of the α-helical domains is mediated by LOX via a copper-dependent oxidative deamination of lysine side chains followed by condensation to form desmosine and isodesmosine crosslinks [41]. These crosslinks stabilize the elastin structure. β-sheets on the other hand is formed as a result of Gly-Gly and Leu-Val interactions [43]. Both α-helical and β-sheets are energetically favorable conformations. Therefore, the elastin molecule in its natural state assumes a random coil structure that continually transitions between these two states. The random coil structure also exhibits high entropy and upon stretch the molecules align [43]. The extent of stretch is limited by the crosslinks however, it can reach up to 220% of their original length [42] as shown in **Figure 5** above. The architecture of elastin is tissue specific [44] as shown in **Figure 6** below. For instance, elastic fibers are organized into concentric rings of fenestrated elastic lamellae around the arterial lumen alternating with a ring of smooth muscle cells [45], highly branched long fibers in alveoli of lungs

[40], perforated sheets within skin [46] and randomly arranged fibers interspersed with collagen fibers in elastic and articular cartilage [45].

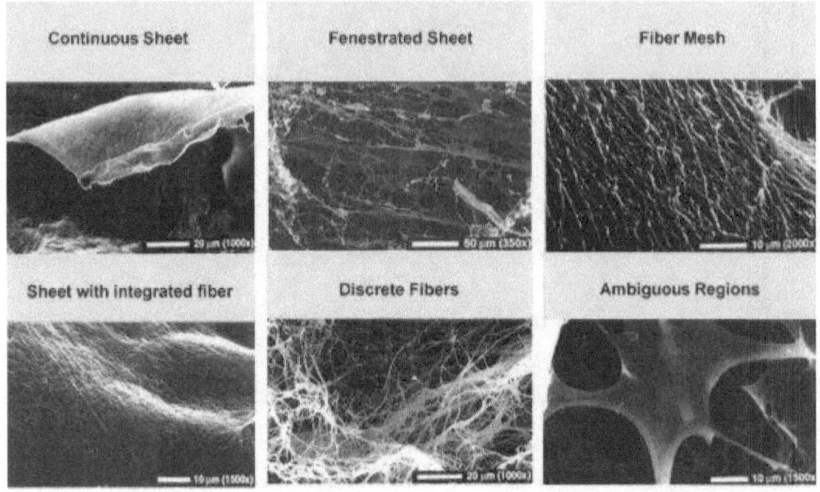

Figure 6: Electron micrographs showing various elastin architectures

2.4.3 Elastin homeostasis and turnover

The cyclic process of synthesis and breakdown of elastin and elastic matrix structures is called elastin homeostasis or elastin remodeling [35] and the rate of breakdown of elastin and its replacement is called elastin turnover [47]. Elastin homeostasis/turnover is an integral part of tissue remodeling as in vascular remodeling or lung fibrosis. As mentioned earlier in **section 2.2.2**, elastin is highly stable under normal circumstances with very limited turn over [33]. The half-life of elastin is almost equivalent to human-life span ~ 70 years as shown in **Figure 7** [48]. However, when subjected to disease or inflammatory microenvironment, elastin becomes susceptible to degradation by proteolytic ('protein degrading') enzymes [33].The most common class of proteolytic enzymes are called Matrix metalloproteinases (MMPs) [49]. Mainly four

MMPs (MMP-2, MMP-7, MMP-9, and MMP-12) have been found in AAA related elastolytic activity [50]. All these MMPs are secreted by macrophages infiltering a site of tissue trauma and cause elastic fiber degradation and inflammation [51]. MMP-2 and MMP-9 are also produced by diseased vascular smooth muscle cells (VSMCs) and are able to activate latent TGF-β [52]. The posttranslational regulation of MMP activity happens at three levels. Initially, MMPs are secreted as inactive pro-MMPs that require proteolytic cleavage of the propeptide. Activity of MMPs is also turned on by the deactivation of a cysteine switch and MMPs are regulated by their specific endogenous inhibitors called tissue inhibitors of metalloproteinase (TIMPs) [53]. Under normal physiological conditions, MMP regulation occurs in transcription level followed by activation of precursor zymogens, interaction with ECM components and inhibition by its specific inhibitors known as Tissue Inhibitors of Matrix Metalloproteinases or TIMPs [54], [55]. This normal regulation of MMPs and TIMPs get perturbed in inflammatory conditions like arthritis, cancer, atherosclerosis, aneurysms, etc. causing increases in elastin degradation vs. synthesis, since natural synthesis of elastin is nearly non-existential after 16 years of age [56]. Cysteine proteases are another class of proteases involved in the major events in the pathogenesis in abdominal aortic aneurysms. They contribute to transmigration of smooth muscle cells through the elastic lamina, formation of macrophage foam cells, apoptosis of vascular cells and macrophages and plaque rupture [57]. Protein levels of Cathepsins K, L and S (CatK, CatL and CatS) have been found to increase in human AAAs whereas their natural inhibitors, cystatin C have been found to be decreased [58]–[61]. CatK and CatS are expressed by macrophages and SMCs [61] whereas CatL expression is mostly localized in macrophage-rich areas and is low in SMCs [58]. In an elastase infused mouse AAA model, however CatC (a lysosomal protease required for post translational processing of serine proteases) is overexpressed [62]. Gene knockdown of CatC has shown to slow

AAA growth and reduce inflammatory response in elastase infused mice [63].

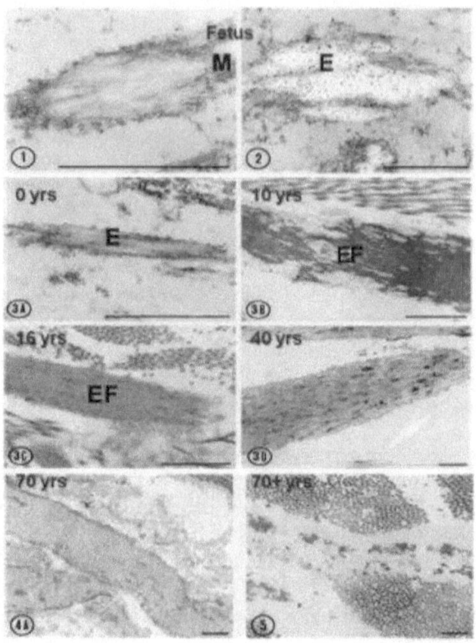

Figure 7: Electron micrographs of elastin fiber homeostasis occurring over years. (1), (2) shows elastic fiber development at fetal stage; 3(A, B, C) shows maturation of elastic fibers during neonatal period; (3A, 4A, 5) shows slow degradation of elastin fibers with age

2.4.4   Abnormalities of the elastic matrix

Elastic fibers are a primary component of elastic tissues like blood vessels, lungs and skin where they impart tissue resilience and elastic stretch and recoil [33]. Therefore, elastin abnormalities have major implications in these organs. Elastin abnormalities include altered amount of elastin, improper fiber assembly, fragmentation of fibers as well as their modification. Elastin abnormalities are both genetic and acquired and further divided into primary elastinopathies (primary defect in fiber assembly) and secondary elatinopathies (disorders in transport and delivery)

[64]. Supravalvular aortic stenosis (SVAS) is an example of primary genetic elastinopathy that occurs as a result of a null mutation in the elastin gene [65]. It is a congenital defect wherein the LV outflow tract is obstructed. The defect is defined by a lesion in the aorta at the sinotubular junction. VSMC hypertrophy, increased collagen and reduced or disorganized elastic fibers in the medial layer contributes to this lesion [65]. **Table II** below summarizes some common elastinopathies.

Table II : List of some common elastinopathies and their features

Disease	Genetic/ Acquired	Features	Reference
Autosomal dominant cutis laxa-1	Genetic	- Frameshift mutation within the last 5 exons of *ELN*. Loss and fragmentation of elastin - loose and hyperextenible skin with redundant fold. - May be accompanied by dilatation of aorta, pulmonary emphysema.	[66], [67]
Marfan Syndrome	Genetic	- Mutation in *FBN1* gene. Abnormalities in elastin-associated microfibrils and increase tissue level of TGFβ and break down of elastin. - Proximal aortic aneurysm, ocular lens dislocation, overgrown long bones.	[68], [69]
Hypertension and arterial stiffening	Acquired	- Occurs in conjunction with diseases associated with defects in elastin and elastic fibers. - Reduced amount of elastin or compromised fiber assembly, altered ECM composition, etc. causes arterial stiffening and leading to hypertension and other complications.	[70]·[71], [72]

Atherosclerosis	Acquired	- Production of tropoelastin, metalloproteases and cathepsins by macrophages. - Degradation of elastic fibers, infiltration of lipids and immune cells into the aortic wall forming plaque.	[73]–[76]
Pseudoxanthoma elasticum	Genetic	- Mutation in ELN gene with largely unknown mechanism. - Pleomorphic elastic fibers, calcification and accumulation in the dermis. - Inelastic skin and cardiovascular abnormalities.	[29]
Aortic Aneurysm and Dissection	Acquired	- Degradation and fragmentation of elastic fibers or improper elastic fiber deposition in the arterial wall of either thoracic or abdominal aorta - Might also occur due to mutation in elastic fiber assembly gene like Lysyl Oxidase (*LOX*) or fibulin (*FBLN*).	[77]–[80]

2.5 Aorta: The major blood vessel

2.5.1 Aortal Structure

2.5.1.1 Gross Anatomy

The aorta is the major artery of the human body which carries blood away from heart to the rest of the body. Blood circulates through the aorta when it leaves the heart and connects with other major arteries to deliver oxygen-rich blood to the brain,

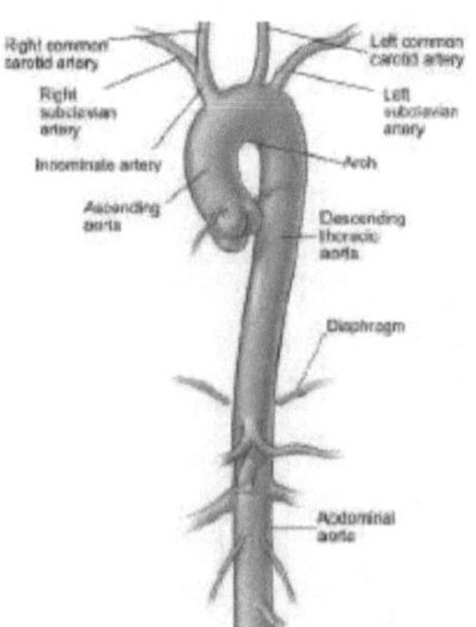

Figure 8: Gross anatomy of the aorta

muscles and other parts of the body [81]. The different parts of the aorta are described below:

2.5.1.1.1 Aortic root

Aortic root is the part of aorta that is attached to the heart. It has aortic valve that allows blood to flow from heart to rest of the body when open and prevents the backflow of blood to heart when closed. The aortic root supplies blood to the heart through left and right coronary arteries [81].

2.5.1.1.2 Ascending aorta

It is the section of aorta which starts at the sinotubular junction of the aortic root and extends up and out from heart and connects with the aortic arch [81].

2.5.1.1.3 Aortic arch

It is the arch shaped part of the aorta which connects the ascending aorta with the descending aorta. The major arteries branching off from aortic arch are brachiocephalic artery (supplies blood to the right arm and right side of the brain), left carotid artery (supplies left side of the brain) and left subclavian artery (supplies blood to the left arm) [81].

2.5.1.1.4 Descending thoracic aorta

It begins at the end of the aortic arch and runs down to the abdomen. Descending aorta is further divided into 2 parts. Thoracic aorta and abdominal aorta. Thoracic aorta continues from aortic arch to the diaphragm. It supplies blood to the muscles of the chest wall and spinal cord [81].

2.5.1.1.5   Abdominal aorta

The aorta continues to descend from the diaphragm to the iliac bifurcation just above the pelvis. There are 5 major branches of the abdominal aorta : celiac artery (supplies to the stomach, liver and pancreas), the superior mesenteric artery (supplies to the small intestine), the inferior mesenteric artery (supplies to the large intestine) and the renal arteries (supplies to the kidneys, muscles in the abdominal wall and lower spinal cord). The iliac bifurcation supplies blood to the legs and the pelvic organs [81].

2.5.1.2 Histology

Histologically, the aorta is divided into three distinct layers: tunica intima, tunica media and tunica adventitia as shown in **Figure 9.**

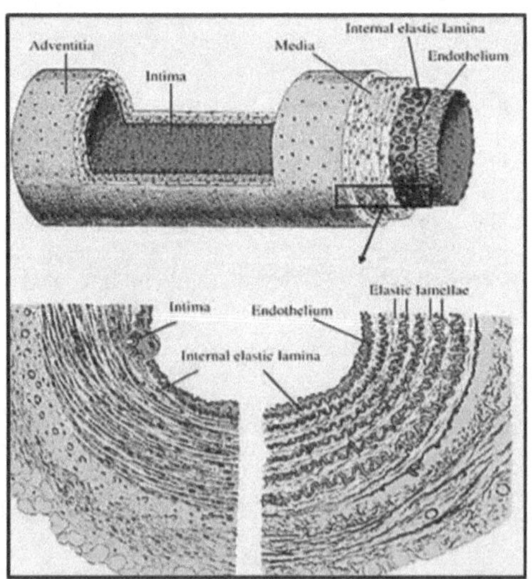

Figure 9: Structural layers of the aorta

2.5.1.2.1   Tunica Intima

It is the innermost lining of the aorta wall and is composed of a monolayer of endothelial cells that provides protection against thrombosis [82]. Endothelial cells secret specific molecules like nitric oxide and inhibit platelet activation and thrombus formation [83], [84]. It also helps in exchanging nutrients and gases specially in capillaries which only has intimal layer. It is separated from medial layer by internal elastic lamellae [85]. In diseases like dissection, the intima is separated from adventitia creating a false lumen [83]. Similarly, in atherosclerosis, the intimal layer is injured resulting in thickening, calcification and ulceration of the intima [83].

2.5.1.2.2   Tunica Adventitia

It is the outermost layer of the aorta wall. It is mainly composed of collagenous extracellular matrix and fibroblast cells [82]. It also contains nerve supply and vasa vasorum (the network of microvessels) that supplies nutrients and oxygen to the aorta wall [86]. Due to higher collagen content, adventitia has higher tensile strength compared to other layers of aorta [85]. The primary function of adventitia is to protect the vessel from excessive extension and ultimate burst upon encountering high pressure of blood [81].

2.5.1.2.3   Tunica Media

The tunica media is the middle layer of the aorta wall. It consists of the concentric ring of SMCs and is separated from intima and adventitia by concentric rings of elastic fibers, called the internal and external elastic lamellae [82]. Elastin molecules are synthesized by SMCs and are incorporated into elastic fibers [82]. The elastic lamellae help the artery to maintain blood pressure while withstanding variations in hemodynamic stress of the cardiac systole and diastole [87].

VSMCs present in the medial layer possess a unique characteristic of phenotypic switching. They assume a quiescent contractile phenotype under normal physiological condition and controls the dilation and contraction of blood vessels hence regulating the blood flow [88]. However, under pathological conditions they switch to a synthetic, non-contractile phenotype characterized by increased cell proliferation and increased matrix production [88], [89]. VSMCs also respond to variety of biochemical and biomechanical signals in the dynamic arterial wall environment leading to change in their function and phenotype [88], [89]. They also transmit the signals to the matrix via cell surface receptors which connects the external environment to the cytoskeleton [90]. The extracellular matrix surrounding the VSMCs also sequesters and releases the biochemical signal [82]. The phenotypic switching and ECM production are also dependent on these signals which are mediated by cell-elastic fiber contact [82]. Hence the arterial structure is stabilized by elastic fibers via regulation of proliferation, phenotypic modulation and VSMCs organization [91], [92].

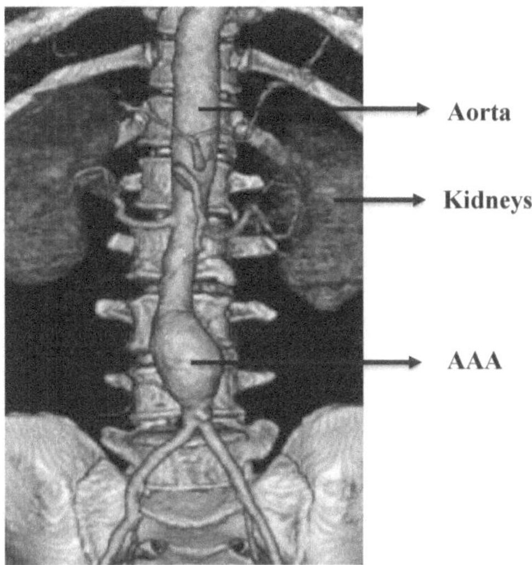

Figure 10: Abdominal aortic aneurysm (AAA)

AAAs are localized, focal dilatations of the abdominal aorta, the segment between the renal bifurcation and iliac bifurcation. Increase in diameter of abdominal aorta at least one and half times the average normal diameter is defined as AAA [93]. Thus, an abdominal aortic segment of maximal diameter > 3.0 cm is considered as aneurysmal [94]. In US, the prevalence of AAA ranges from 0.5% to 3.2% in autopsy studies whereas a large screening study found the prevalence to be 1.4% [95]. Death due to ruptured AAAs in the United States is estimated to be 15,000 per year making it the 13th leading cause of death nationally [95]. Increased incidence of AAAs ranges from 4.2% to 11% per year globally has been reported by epidemiological studies [96]–[99]. The risk factors for occurrence of AAAs include age, sex, ethnicity, smoking and genetic predispositions as well as conditions like hypertension [93]. AAAs has high incidence in Caucasian males above 60 years of age [93]. The risk is even higher in people who are smokers or have ever smoked [93]. Similarly, people with other pre-existing conditions like atherosclerosis, hypertension as well as family history are found to be at greater risk of getting aneurysms [100]. The risk of rupture on the other hand depends on aneurysm size (highest risk on aneurysm > 5.5cm diameter), the expansion rate, continued smoking, uncontrolled hypertension and increased wall stress [50].

2.6.1 Pathophysiology of AAA: Cellular and molecular mechanisms

AAAs are multifactorial conditions that involve breakdown and loss of aortal wall ECM structures resulting in gradual wall thinning and weakening and ultimate rupture [101]–[104]. Histological analyses of human AAA tissues show infiltration of leukocyte, degradation of extracellular matrix and depletion and apoptosis of VSMCs to be the major pathological hallmarks of AAA which has also been recapitulated by histological study of elastase infused rodent AAA models [105]–[108]. Although the exact mechanism of the disease is not clearly understood, studies on animal models of the disease have shown the involvement of local inflammatory responses; this incites infiltration of inflammatory and immune cells (macrophages, neutrophils, mast cells, T and B lymphocytes) [108], [109], which is further enhanced by various cytokines and extracellular matrix proteases (mostly MMP-9) to cause VSMC apoptosis and ECM degradation with loss of aortic wall integrity [110]. In other words, the destructive pathological remodeling of aorta in AAA involves four interrelated factors: (a) chronic inflammation of the outer wall of aorta along with neovascularization and upregulation of proinflammatory cytokines (b) hyper production and dysregulation of matrix degrading enzymes, (c) progressive destruction of elastin and collagen and (d) apoptosis of medial smooth muscle cells (SMCs) resulting in impaired capacity for connective tissue repair. **Figure 11** below shows a series of processes involved in the formation of AAAs. In response to any adverse stimuli like chronic hypertension, atherosclerosis, smoking or vasculitis; recruitment of inflammatory cells to the medial and adventitial layer of aorta and upregulation of matrix degrading MMPs (mainly MMP-9) appears to be the initial crucial step which is followed by breaking down of elastic matrix and generation of elastin degradation products (EDPs) or elastin peptides [111], [112]. Matrix degradation can further release chemoattractant molecules which amplify and recruit more inflammatory cells to the aorta wall as well as causes apoptosis of SMCs [111].

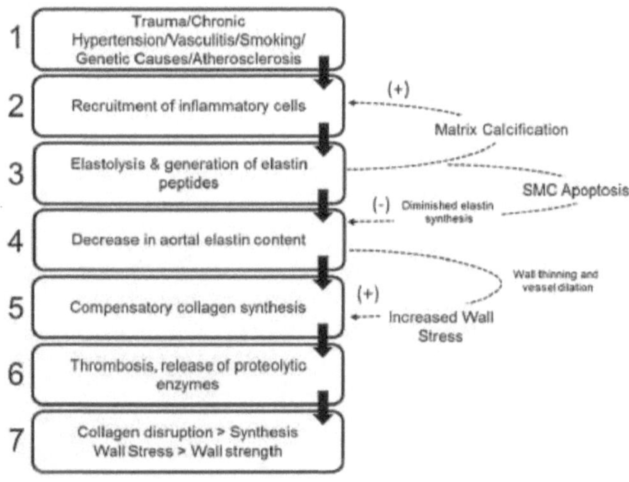

Figure 11: AAA disease etiology

The decrease in total aortal elastin content due to upregulated MMP-9 is compensated by deposition of collagen [113]. Unlike elastin which has very limited production and fiber formation capability in later stage of life, collagen is readily deposited by adult VSMCs and fibroblasts [113]. Continued degradation of elastin leads to aortal wall thinning, loss of stretch and recoil properties and increased wall stress due to blood flow. There is increased perception of blood flow stresses by VSMCs which responds by increasing compensatory collagen synthesis. The compensatory mechanism stabilizes the weakened aorta wall for short term causing slow growth of AAA (5 to 7 years) before rupture [114], [115]. However, the continued degradation of elastin and generation of elastin peptides activates SMC apoptosis and provides positive stimulus for collagen breakdown as described previously in **section 2.4.4** and in **Figure 11** [116]. Eventually, an imbalance between collagen synthesis and collagen breakdown results, causing increased in wall stress and susceptibility of the aortal wall to fatal hemodynamic stress-induced rupture [111]. Therefore, breaking the chain of events early by attenuating elastolysis and promoting new elastic fiber regeneration in the aortal wall can be a potential approach to slow or regress AAA growth.

2.6.2   Histological characteristics of AAAs

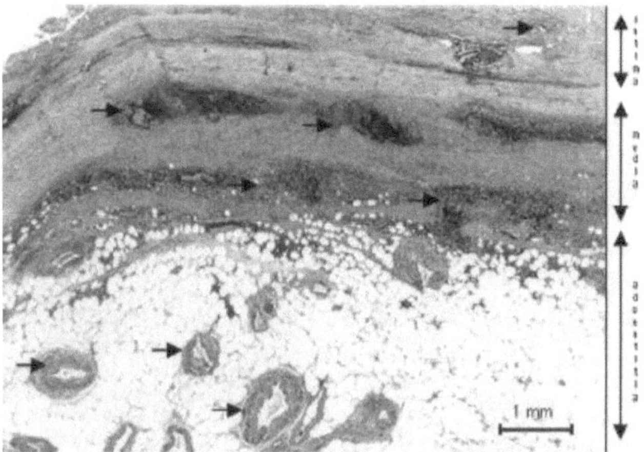

Figure 12: Movat's pentachrome staining showing thickening of intima, scarcity of medial elastic fibers and SMCs and dense cellular infiltrates in the adventitia and media-adventitia transition in human AAA tissue

Studies have shown complete distortion of the aortic wall structure with complete disorganization of internal and external elastic laminae and the landmarks of intimal-medial and medial-adventitial transition as shown in **Figure 12**. Hellenthal et.al. have carried out a detailed study of the tissues obtained from thirty-nine AAA patients with elective or emergency aneurysm repair surgery. A mean maximal diameter of 67mm and a mean growth rate of 6mm/year [117].

They found complete loss of endothelial cells in the intimal layer as revealed by CD31-CD34 staining. The original intima was shifted to the intraluminal side of the remnants of the internal elastic laminae [117]. They also found a thickened intimal layer with fibrin and cholesterol clefts as well as presence of sporadic macrophages on the intima-intra luminal thrombus (ILT) transitional zone. The medial layer was characterized by limited elastin content with fragmented and distorted elastin structure. The abdominal aorta wall also infiltrated by T lymphocytes and to a lesser extent by macrophages. Regions with a higher number of T-lymphocytes exhibited lower elastin content. Regions surrounding the inflammatory cell infiltrates were particularly devoid of SMCs, possibly due to apoptotic loss. There was increased microvessel density in the outer media and adventitia. Collagen was characterized by thin fibrils on the luminal side and thick fibrils on the adventitial side of the media. This finding was also echoed in other studies which showed cholesterol crystal laden intima with medial atrophy,

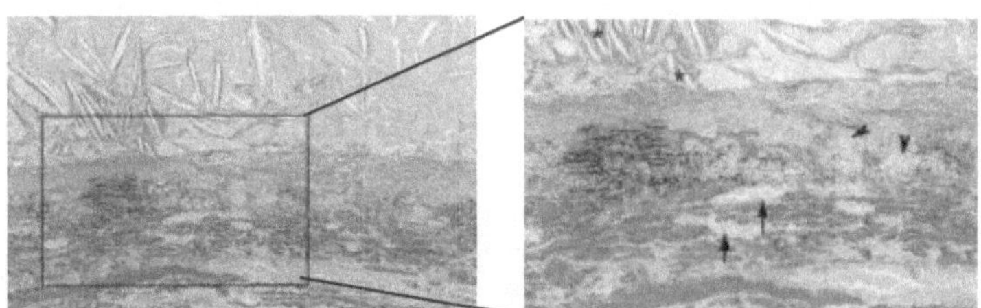

Figure 13: VVG stained section of 60 years old make AAA patient's abdominal aorta showing cholesterol crystal laden intima and atrophy of media

fragmented elastin and progressive thickening of adventitia with expanded network of vasa vasorum as shown in **Figure 13** [118].

This expanded network of vasa vasora contributes to recruitment of inflammatory cells that is found in aneurysmal wall. These cells secret cytotoxic mediators that cause SMC apoptosis [119]. These cells also secrete chemoattractant to further attract more inflammatory cells thereby causing chronic inflammation and continued matrix degradation [50].

2.7   Current diagnosis and treatment of AAA

AAAs are mostly asymptomatic and detected incidentally with ultrasonography (USG), Computed Tomography (CT) scanning or Magnetic Resonance Imaging (MRI) performed for other indications [120]. Various guidelines have been issued for screening AAAs for early detection like The United States Preventive Services Task Force (USPSTF) guidelines, The American College of Cardiology/American Heart Association (ACC/AHA) guidelines and the Canadian Society for Vascular Surgery guidelines all of which recommend at least one time screening using ultrasonography of males above 65 years of age who have ever smoked [120].

2.8 Current management of AAAs

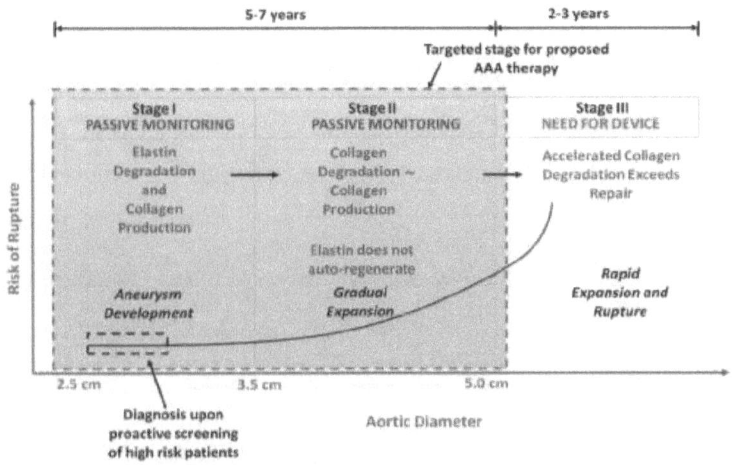

Figure 14: Schematic showing current management of AAA

Currently no treatment exists for small AAAs (< 5.5 cm maximal aortal diameter) except routine screening of high-risk patient using ultrasound or CT **(Figure 14)**. Early surgical intervention does not appear to improve the long-term survivability of patients. Hence no active treatment currently exists for small AAAs [121]. The gradual increase of aortic diameter takes place over period of 5 to 7 years after which the aorta reaches the rupture stage (5.5 cm diameter) [114], [115]. Upon reaching this stage, the aneurysm is surgically fixed **(Figure 15)**. Before the 1990s, open repair was the only surgical treatment option available for AAAs. In open repair, the aneurysmal segment of the aorta is surgically removed and replaced with synthetic vascular graft [122]. It is a highly invasive procedure and unsuitable for elderly patients to withstand. Although open repair provides immediate solution to the survivors, it is associated with higher perioperative morbidity and mortality [121]. Surgical risks include major hemorrhage, multiple organ dysfunction syndrome (MODS) related to reperfusion injury following aortic clamping [123]. A better alternative to open surgical repair is an elective intervention called Endovascular Repair (EVAR). EVAR provides several benefits over open repair like it is minimally invasive and reportedly has reduced post-operative mortality and morbidity [124]. EVAR also has reduced risk of reperfusion injury and MODS and is suitable for patients with several comorbidities who cannot withstand open repair [124]. In EVAR, a fabric covered stent inserted into the catheter is guided through an artery in the groin to the abdominal aortaand then released. The stent graft provides a clear lumen in the aneurysmal segment to restores blood flow [122].

Despite having several benefits over open repair, endovascular repair is also accompanied by several complications like surrounding blood vessel damage, renal failure, endoleak or continual leaking of blood from graft into the aneurysm sac with potential rupture, groin hematoma, intimal hyperplasia etc. [117]. Also, not all patients are suitable for endovascular repair [117]. Therefore, the complications associated with both the repair methods and assessment of their risk to benefit invokes the critical need

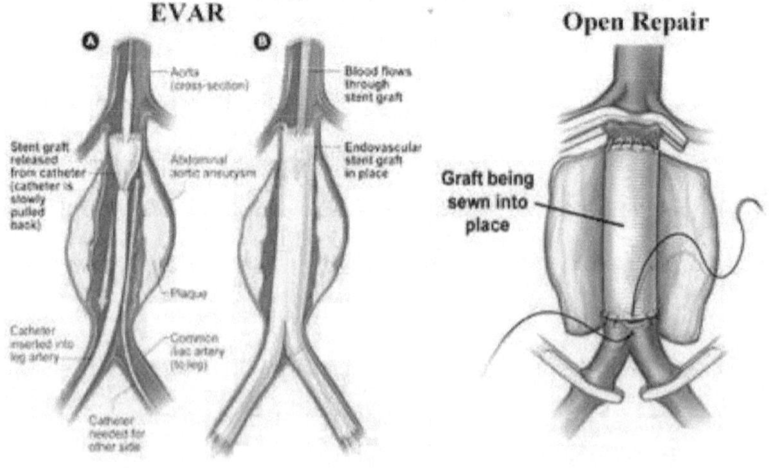

of alternative, minimally invasive treatments to arrest or regress small AAAs during their years-long growth to a critical size.

2.9   Strategies to attenuate or arrest AAA growth

AAAs are often asymptomatic and characterized by three distinct histopathological regions: inflammatory, active and amorphous, each of which are characterized by cellular components and ECM architecture [110]. A large number of inflammatory cells are frequently localized on the adventitial side of the media in the inflammatory region. These cells include T and B cells, macrophages, mast cells and neutrophils, all of which secrete proinflammatory cytokines and drive chronic inflammation [110]. The active region is characterized by increases in matrix degrading enzymes like MMP-9, decrease in VSMCs and destruction of elastic lamellae of the aorta wall. The maximally dilated area of the AAA is characterized by tissue containing some amorphous elastin and abundant fibro-collagenous ECM [110]. While surgical intervention or endovascular repair is mandated only at the pre-rupture stage, AAAs inevitably progresses gradually with an increase in rupture risk [110]. Hence an effective strategy to attenuate AAA growth has long been desired. To accomplish this, intensive studies are being pursued to identify the genetic and molecular mechanisms of AAA so as to develop therapies aimed at attenuating AAA growth in the years preceding their assumption of rupture-prone dimensions. Some of the therapeutic targets being investigated for attenuation of AAA growth are summarized below:

2.9.1 Pro-inflammatory mediators

Pro-inflammatory mediators are one of the most important players in the progression of AAAs. These are biological factors that shift the balance of ECM metabolism towards tissue degradation by activating inflammatory signaling pathways. Several pro-inflammatory mediators like TNF-α and monocyte chemoattractant factor-1 (MCP-1) have been implicated in the pathogenesis of AAAs [50]. These mediators are known to cause and maintain the inflammatory response by inducing inflammatory cell infiltration. Most proinflammatory mediators activate signaling molecules like c-Jun N-terminal kinase (JNK) and nuclear factor-κB (NF- κB) and these activated signaling pathways enhance the expression of pro-inflammatory mediators thus causing the vicious cycle of chronic inflammation [110]. Pro-inflammatory signaling pathways also activate ECM degradation enzymes like MMP-9 and MMP-2 while reducing the expression of enzymes like lysyl oxidase (LOX) that are critical to crosslinking of elastic fibers and collagen fibers [110]. This causes an overall loss of stability of elastic fibers, their degradation and loss, to result in AAA growth. Several pharmacotherapies are thus being explored for targeted suppression of pro-inflammatory mediators, modulation of intracellular signaling pathways, and inhibition ECM degradation. Some of the recent pharmacotherapies are listed in **Table III** below:

Table III. List of some common pharmacotherapies and their mechanism of AAA inhibition

Drug	Target	Model	Mechanism of AAA inhibition	Reference
α-Tocopherol (vitamin E)	Oxidative stress	ATII/ApoE$^{-/-}$ mice Elastase infused rat	↓ ROS, ↓ macrophage infiltration	[125], [126]
Doxycycline	MMP	Elastase infused rats/mice, $CaCl_2$	↓ MMP-9, Elastin preservation	[110]

		mice, ATII/ApoE$^{-/-}$ mice		
ACE inhibitor	RAS	Elastase rat	Elastin preservation	[127]
ARB	RAS	Elastase rat	↓ Macrophage infiltration, ↓ NF-κB activity, ↓ MMP-9	[127]
Statin	Mevalonate pathway	Elastase mice, Elastase rat, Elastase/ApoE$^{-/-}$ mice	↓ Macrophage infiltration, ↓ NF-κB activity, ↓ MMP-9, ↓ MCP-1, elastin preservation	[110][128], [129]
SP600125	JNK	CaCl$_2$ mice, ATII/ApoE$^{-/-}$ mice	↓ Macrophage infiltration, ↓ MMP-9, elastin preservation, regression of established AAA	[110]

2.9.2   Intracellular signaling pathways

Many intracellular signaling pathways have been implicated in AAA initiation and progression. Once such aberrant signaling pathway involves the cytokine, transforming growth factor-beta (TGF-β). Studies have shown that systemic blockade of TGF-β or removal of SMAD3 gene which is a downstream signal of TGF-β, causes augmentation of Angiotensin II (Ang II)- and CaCl$_2$-induced AAAs [130]. TGF- β signaling occurs at multiple levels with diverse functions, but in general, TGF-β1 binds to TGF-β1 type II receptor and activates the SMAD signaling pathway [131]. Activation of SMAD signaling triggers downstream increases in MMP-2 and MMP-9 expression via SMAD 3 and SMAD 4 mediation respectively [131]. Notch1 is another signaling mediator that has been shown to be increased in both human AAAs and AngII-induced mouse models. Pharmaco-inhibition of Notch 1 or haplosufficiency in the Notch 1 pathway have shown to attenuate the formation of Ang II-induced AAAs in mice by preventing the influx of inflammatory macrophages at the aneurysmal site by causing defects in the macrophage migration and proliferation [132].

Several studies have shown the association of oxidative stress with aneurysm formation in clinical patients as well as in animal models of the disease. Generation of reactive oxygen species (ROS) like the superoxide anion, and hydroxyl radical and reactive nitrogen species like nitric oxide and peroxynitrite have been found to be increased in human AAAs which suggests the potential contribution of ROS to aortic wall degeneration [133]. Inflammatory cytokines like IL-1β, TNF-α and IFN-γ which are upregulated in the aneurysmal milieu are a potential trigger of cellular ROS production in the AAA wall [134]. These proinflammatory cytokines can enhance inducible nitric oxide synthase (iNOS) expression in aortal SMCs which are capable of activating MMPs and inducing apoptosis of SMCs [135]. Other potential sources of ROS include membrane associated NADPH oxidases, xanthine oxidase (XO), etc. produced by vascular cell types during inflammation. ROS promote AAA formation and growth by activating MMPs and inducing apoptosis of aortal SMCs [135]. Hypoxia and hydrogen peroxide can also induce a number of genes like hydrogen peroxide-inducible clone 5 (Hic-5). A study by Lei et al has shown that Hic-5 activates the mitogen activated protein kinase (MAP) c-Jun N-terminal Kinase pathway leading to aneurysm development [136]. Xiong et.al has shown that both pharmacologic inhibition of NADPH oxidase by apomycin as well as iNOS$^{-/-}$ suppress AAA formation. This effect was found to be associated with reduced expression of MMP-2 and MMP-9 and decreased production of nitric oxide metabolite [135]. The decrease in elastolytic MMPs has vital implications to slowing elastic matrix breakdown and thus rat of AAA growth. Even though very limited information is available on the mechanistic aspect, some animal studies have demonstrated the relationship between the renin-angiotensin-aldosterone system (RAAS) and AAA development.

2.9.3   Post-transcriptional regulators

Recent studies have investigated the delivery of microRNAs to modulate the extensive functional networks involved in the complex interactions between cellular-related mechanisms, inflammatory mediators and extracellular matrix degradation in AAA progression. MicroRNAs are small non-coding RNAs which are key post-transcriptional regulators for genes and physiological processes involved in AAA progression. miR-21, miR-24, miR-29b, miR-712 and miR-205 are five microRNAs that have been implicated in AAA development [137]. The different microRNAs act via distinct mechanisms in AAAs and hence their inhibition targets selective factors and processes that contribute to AAA pathology. For instance, reduced aortic dilatation was observed by inhibiting miR-29b in elastase-perfused and AngII-infused mice [138]. Differently, overexpression of miR-21 or miR-24 was found to inhibit AAA development in both the animal models [139], [140]. The differences in the functional effects of overexpressing or inhibiting selected microRNAs on AAAs are related to the downstream gene targets of each specific microRNA [137]. Different members of the miR-29 family, among other miRs have been widely detected to target several key genes and pathways involved in fibrosis and ECM regulation including different collagen isoforms, fibrillin-1 and elastin [141]–[144]. Several studies have reported that TGF-b suppresses miR-29b expression in a SMAD 3 dependent manner (**Figure 16**) increasing collagen synthesis and triggers a pro-fibrotic or protective effect in aneurysm [145] There is also evidence that inhibiting miR-29b with locked nucleic acid

(LNA)-anti-miR-29b upregulates collagen and elastin genes and in parallel downregulates MMP-2 and MMP-9 in two independent mouse AAA models, the porcine pancreatic elastase (PPE) infusion-injury model and the AngII/ApoE$^{-/-}$ mouse model [138]. Differently, overexpressing miR-29b using lentiviral vectors caused significant increases in AAA formation and AAA rupture rate [138]·[145].

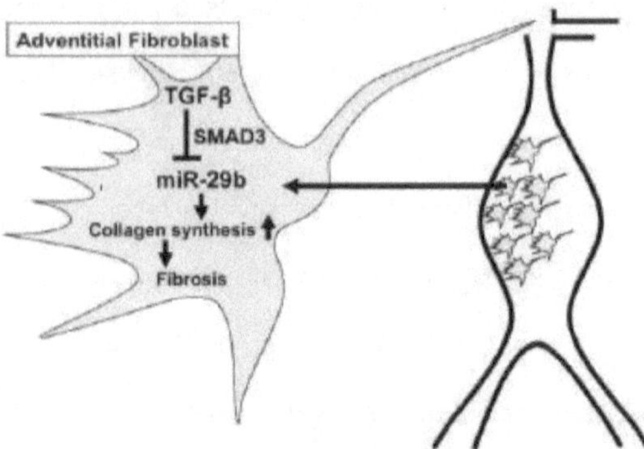

Figure 16: Schematic showing the role and regulation of miR-29b in adventitial fibroblasts during AAA progression

2.9.4   Other Strategies for attenuating AAA growth

Gene silencing using small interfering RNA or siRNA are being widely studied as a promising technology to silence the genes involved in AAA pathogenesis. Like microRNA, siRNA also belongs to the family of small non-coding RNA family. In siRNA therapies, small double-stranded interfering RNAs (siRNAs) are introduced into the cytoplasm [146]–[148]. The siRNAs are complementary to the target mRNA to be silenced and are processed by RNA induced silencing complex (RISC) inside the cytoplasm. The RISC locates the target mRNA using siRNA as template. Once the RISC localized to the target mRNA, the ribonuclease cleaves the target mRNA silencing the gene [149]. This mechanism of action is summarized in **Figure 17** [150].

Some of the recent work involving use of siRNA targeting MMPs and other potential targets for AAAs are summarized below in **Table 4**.

Table IV: Summary of recent work using siRNA for AAAs

Type	Target	Location	Function	Mechanism	Reference
Immune Modulator	Toll-like receptors 2 and 4 (TLR2 and 4)	Macrophage, dendritic cells	Innate immune system, inflammation	↓ NF-κB activity, MCP-1, IL-8 etc. ↓calcification via BMP-2, ↓MMP-2 and MMP-9	[151], [152]
	C-C chemokine receptor type 2 (CCR2)	Vascular cells and immune cells	Monocyte chemotaxis	Disruption of MCP-1/CCR2 signaling pathway	[153]
	S100 alarmins (S100A9 and S100A4)	S100A4 secreted by neutrophils, macrophages, S100A9 expressed in synthetic SMCs	Calcium-binding, cancer metastasis, neutrophil activity stimulation and phagocytosis	↓VSMC proliferation, MMP-2 and MMP-9 expression	[154]
ROS	NADPH oxidase 4 (Nox 4)	Membrane bound enzyme	Generation of radical oxygen species	Adventitial fibroblast activation, ↓adventitial inflammation, IL-6 and MCP-1 secretion	[155]
Transcription factors	Kruppel like factor 4 (KLF4)	Endothelial cells and inflamed SMCs	Regulation of macrophage activation and SMC phenotype switching	Attenuation of downregulation of smooth muscle marker gene expression, SMC	[156]

				differentiati on	
Metalloprotein ases (MMPs)	MMP-2/MMP-9/MMP-12	Aneurysmal smooth muscle cells, endothelial cells, macrophage	ECM remodeling , migration, remodeling	MMP-2: ↓SMC invasion; MMP-9/12: ↓beta-catenin signaling, proliferation via cyclin D1 mechanism	[157]
Protein Kinase	Extracellu lar signal -regulated kinases 1/2 (ERK 1/2)	MAPK family	Proliferatio n and differentiat ion of different cells including VSMCs, MMP activation	↓MMP2 formation in AAA	[158]
	JNK, JNK 2	MAPK family	Cellular stress signaling, cell apoptosis	JNK1 or 2: ↓MMP activity, JNK1 and 2 combined: ↓all MMP activity	[159]
	Protein Kinase B (AKT)	Serine/threo nine protein kinase	Modulatio n of apoptosis, proliferatio n, migration, etc., abnormal vascular remodeling	↓proMMP-9 , proMMP-2 and active MMP-2, ↑TIMP-1 activity	[160]

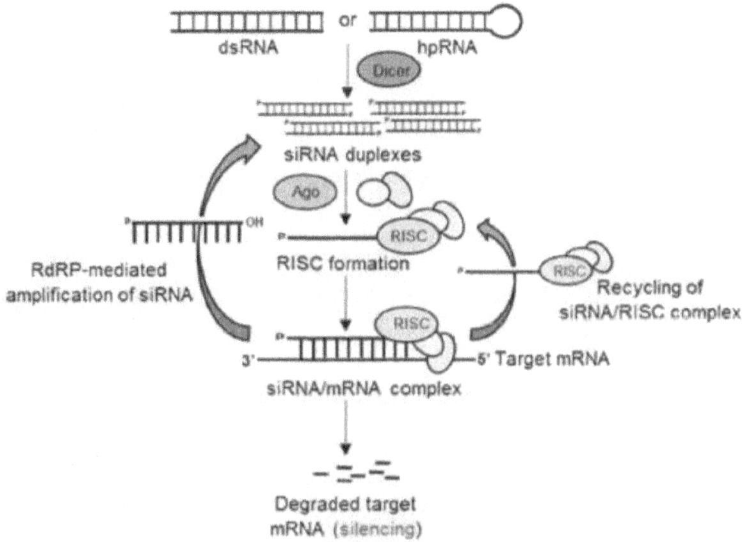

Figure 17: Schematics of RNAi-mediated gene silencing in eukaryotes

Even though gene silencing using siRNA has demonstrated promising outcomes in both *in vitro* and preclinical animal studies, significant challenges remain that need to be addressed. These include tissue specificity of siRNA effects, target/sequence validation, transfection efficiency and unwanted off-target safety concerns. Another major limitation of this technology is the very short half-life of siRNAs *in vivo* [161]. To address these issues, siRNA delivery systems such as nanoparticles are being investigated.

Nanoparticles are capable of overcoming the challenges and barriers associated with delivery of therapeutic agents particularly, biodistribution and bioavailability. They ensure predictable and steady bioavailability of delivered therapeutics in the tissue of interest and limit their systemic biodistribution in other organs. They provide superior *in vivo* retention by (i) decreasing enzymatic degradation of therapeutics and (ii) protecting against sequestration by phagocytes of the reticulo-endothelial systems. The improved localization of nanoparticles in the diseased vascular wall can also result from enhanced permeability of the compromised vasculature [162]. Besides siRNA, nanoparticles have also been extensively investigated for targeted delivery of therapeutics to injured or diseased blood vessels as in AAAs. For instance, Camardo et.al investigated the sustained and steady release of doxycycline (DOX) from PEG-PLGA nanoparticles to inhibit JNK 2 in order to impart pro-elastogenic and anti-proteolytic effects to AAAs [163]. Their study suggested the pro-matrix regenerative benefit was imparted by the combined effect of DOX and cationic-functionalized nanoparticles. Another study by Fox et.al demonstrated successful targeting of cathepsin K conjugated DOX loaded PLGA submicron particles to the aneurysmal site to impart anti-proteolytic and pro-elastogenic benefits [164].

2.10 Cell Therapy: Potential Alternative Strategy for Elastic Matrix Regeneration

Almost all elastin regenerative repair strategies explored so far are focused on reversing or attenuating adverse signaling pathways or mitigating MMP overexpression in the AAA wall, with limited or no direct emphasis on addressing either poor elastogenesis and matrix regeneration and repair. Even though healthy adult VSMCs have limited elastogenic capacity and diseased SMCs like that in AAAs are even more non-elastogenic, studies have demonstrated the reversibility of SMC activation in the presence of growth factors and other biomolecular and environmental cues promoting the contractile SMC phenotype [165]. For e.g. Ramamurthi et.al have shown the *in vitro* benefits of HA oligomer and exogenous TGF-β in enhancing the elastin synthesis and fiber formation in both healthy as well as diseased rat and human VSMCs [166]–[168]. Cell therapy is one of the potent strategies that has the potential to address the challenges of other regenerative strategies by providing dual benefit of anti-proteolysis and pro-elastogenicity. Cell therapy can provide miRNA, produce a range of proelastogenic signaling cues, reduce MMP expression and also likely to have fewer ethical and technical concerns compared to other techniques like gene delivery [169]·[138]. Studies have shown to reduce the MMP activity and promote stabilization of AAAs by endovascular delivery of syngeneic vascular SMCs in rat model however, no effect was seen in terms of elastic matrix regeneration and AAA regression [170]. Hence, introduction of highly elastogenic, autologous cell types might be more effective and clinically translatable to achieve (a) enhanced elastogenesis, (b) suppressed elastolysis, (c) localized, controlled, predictable and sustained delivery of therapeutics, (c) improve ability of AAA SMCs to crosslink elastin precursors into matrix structures and (d) promote elastic matrix synthesis by elastogenically induced AAA cells[166]. However, no such clinically approved cell therapy currently exists.

2.11 Stem cells

Stem cells represent a unique population of undifferentiated cells which are capable of extensively differentiating into different tissue and cell types. They are characterized by (i) self-renewal, (ii) clonality and (iii) potency. However, their properties might vary depending on the type of stem cells [171]. For instance, embryonic stem cells (ESCs) are more potent and have greater ability of self-renewal compared to adult stem cells (ASCs) [171]. Stem cells are normally classified based on differentiation potential and their origin [172].

2.11.1 Classification based on potency

2.11.1.1 Totipotent stem cells

These are the cells found in early development and are most undifferentiated. These cells have capacity to differentiate into three primary germ layers of the embryo as well as to develop the extra embryonic tissues like placenta. For e.g. fertilized ootcyte is totipotent cells [173].

2.11.1.2 Pluripotent Stem Cells

Pluripotent stem cells can differentiate into cells of all three germ layers. Most common pluripotent stem cells are Embryonic Stem Cells (ECS) [174].

2.11.1.3 Multipotent Stem Cells

Multipotent stem cells are present in most tissues. They mostly differentiate into cells from a single germ layer. Mesenchymal Stem Cells (MSCs) are the most common cells of this category which are adherent to cell culture plastics, characterized by specific cell surface markers and can differentiate into cells that formt he parenchyma of tissues of mesodermal origin like adipose tissue, bone, cartilage and muscle. Some recent studies have also shown the trans differentiation of MSCs into neuronal tissues which are ectodermal in origin [175], [176].

2.11.1.4 Oligopotent Stem Cells

Oligopotent stem cells can form 2 or more lineages within a specific tissue. For e.g. oligopotent stem cells present in the ocular surface and cornea of the pig can generate individual colonies of corneal and conjunctival cells [177]. Hematopoietic stem cells are the most commonly known oligopotent stem cells which can differentiate into both myeloid and lymphoid lineages [178].

2.11.1.5 Unipotent Stem Cells

As the name suggests, these cells can differentiate into only one specific cell type from a single lineage. For e.g. muscle stem cells differentiate into only mature muscle cells and type II pneumocyte of alveoli give rise to type I pneumocytes [179]–[182].

2.11.2 Classification based on origin:

2.11.2.1 Embryonic Stem Cells

ESCs are pluripotent stem cells derived from the inner cell mass of the blastocyst. They can differentiate into cells of the three primary germ layers [183]. These cells retain their undifferentiated state for a long time in culture though the culture conditions play critical role on their ability to maintain this state [184]. These cells are characterized by the presence of transcription factors like Nanog, and Oct 4 [185], [186]. These cells are excellent tool to understand human development and organogenesis. Their unlimited proliferation and pluripotency provide remarkable access to tissues from human body and support basic research on the differentiation and function of human tissues and also provide materials for testing the safety and efficacy of human drugs while avoiding the use of animal models [184]. However, direct use of undifferentiated ESC for tissue transplant can cause teratoma formation or cancer development and ethical concerns of using the embryo to generate these cells limit their use [171].

2.11.2.2 Adult Stem Cells

Stem cells derived from adult tissues include MSCs and human amnion epithelial cells derived from placental tissues [187]. These cells are known for their anti-inflammatory properties as well as tissue repair capabilities [188]. These cells are widely used for cell therapy because autologous implantation of these cells prevent rejection and they also do not raise any ethical concerns in their sourcing and effects upon implantation [188], [189].

2.11.2.3 Tissue-Resident Stem Cells

These type of stem cells are resident in adult tissues and generate tissue specific terminally differentiated cells [190]. These cells are shown to originate during ontogenesis and remain in inactive state until their proliferation, differentiation or migration is activated by local stimuli [191], [192]. They reside in a microenvironment called stem cell niche which controls their self-renewal and differentiation [193]. The niche also plays critical role in stem cell homeostasis and tissue repair through various signals from extracellular matrix and soluble mediators that mediates cell signaling and gene expression [194].

2.11.2.4 Induced Pluripotent Stem Cells

Induced pluripotent stem cells (iPSCs) are produced by genetically reprogramming adult somatic cells to ESC-like state [195]. The first reported iPSCs were produced in 2007 from mouse by transducing mouse fibroblasts with octamer-binding transcription factor ¾ (OCT ¾), SRY-related high mobility group box protein-2 (SOX2), the oncoprotein c-MYC, and Kruppel-like factor 4 (KLF4) [196]. A year later, human iPSCs were produced in a similar way and was shown that these cells were similar to human ESCs in terms of morphology, proliferation, surface antigens, gene expression, epigenetic status of pluripotent cell-specific genes, telomerase activity and their differentiation into cell types of 3 germ layers in culture [196]. iPSCs are widely used to study drug development, disease modelling and regenerative medicine, however, the retroviral vectors used for transfection and oncogenic factors like c-MYC used to reprogram the cells can cause cancer. Studies are being conducted to replace the viral transfection method by non-viral vector approaches like chemical compounds, plasmids, adenovirus, and transposons [197]–[200].

2.11.3 Mesenchymal Stem Cells

Mesenchymal stem cells were first described by Friedenstein et.al in the early 70s and were first isolated from human bone marrow [201]. These are multipotent adult cells with the potential to differentiate into multiple cell types like osteoblasts, chondrocytes, myocytes, adipocytes, etc [202]. Mesenchyme refers to the embryonic loose connective tissue derived from the mesoderm and develops into hematopoietic and connective tissue. These cells are also synonymously called as mesenchymal stromal cells or marrow stromal cells because some researchers argue that "stem cell" label is not always appropriate especially for connective tissue cells forming the scaffold of an organ because they are not capable of differentiating into osteoblasts, chondrocytes or adipocytes [202]. The International Society for Cellular Therapy (ISCT) has specified the criteria to define MSC populations, which include (i) adherence to substrates, (ii) presence of cluster of differentiation like CD 73, CD90, CD105 surface markers and the absence of CD45, CD34, CD14, CD11b, CD79a, CD19 and class II histocompatibility complex antigens, (iii) potential to differentiation towards osteoblast, adipocyte and chondroblast lineages [203]. Apart from these guidelines, researchers have found that the presence of STRO-1 antigen, VCAM 1/CD106 and melanoma cell adhesion molecule/CD146 is useful in defining MSCs because these antigens characterize the adherent cells with high degree of clonogenicity and multidirectional differentiation ability *in vitro*. MSCs are also defined by their niche, which is the microenvironment of the body where these cells reside and maintain an undifferentiated state [204]–[206]. However, the precise location of the niche for MSCs is still not known. Research shows they can be isolated from various tissues of mesodermal origin like bone marrow, cord cells, adipose tissue, molar cells and amniotic fluid. Morphologically, they have small cell body with a few long and thin cell processes. Once fully confluent they assume cobblestone morphology [207].

Most frequently the MSCs are isolated from bone marrow tissues [208]. Marrow tissues consists of a heterogenous group of cells including hematopoietic cells, endothelial cells and granulomonocytic cells, therefore, these marrow stromal cells are subjected to fractionation on a density gradient solution like Ficoll^{TM} which improves the purification strategies followed by low-density plating methods. Mononuclear cells are collected followed by centrifugation and cultured in tissue culture dishes. Nonadherent cells are removed after 24 hours and the adherent cells are cultivated and passaged [208].

2.11.4 Use of MSCs in cell therapies for AAAs and vascular disorders

As discussed above, the poor elastogenicity of adult VSMCs limits their use for cell therapy. Stem cells can overcome the challenges associated with adult VSMCs. Evidences show that neonatal SMCs are far more elastogenic than adult SMCs and vascular elastin is primarily synthesized and matured during fetal and neonatal development in stem cells or progenitor cells rich tissue microenvironments [208]. Deb et.al have shown the deposition of nascent fiber like elastin deposition in the neointima of rat AAA tissue with sparse distribution of fibrillin-1 pre-scaffolds, the glycoprotein structure that helps in crosslinking and organization of amorphous elastin into mature crosslinked fibers **(Figure 18)**. Contrary to this, they also found fibrillin-1/elastin co-localization in the medial layer explaining the aberrant elastic fiber assembly of the neointimal elastin. However, a remarkable finding of this study was the presence of circulating progenitors like SMAA$^+$ cells in the neointima, which were phenotypically different from medial smooth muscle cells, and thus possibly of a different origin but exhibiting the capability of generating significant amount of nascent elastic fibers [209]. Therefore, it would be justifiable to hypothesize that stem cells/progenitor cells or their early differentiated SMC phenotype would be more elastogenic compared to adult AAA SMCs. Moreover, there is a possibility that these cells could also improve the elastogenicity of AAA SMCs through juxtacrine or paracrine signaling [210].

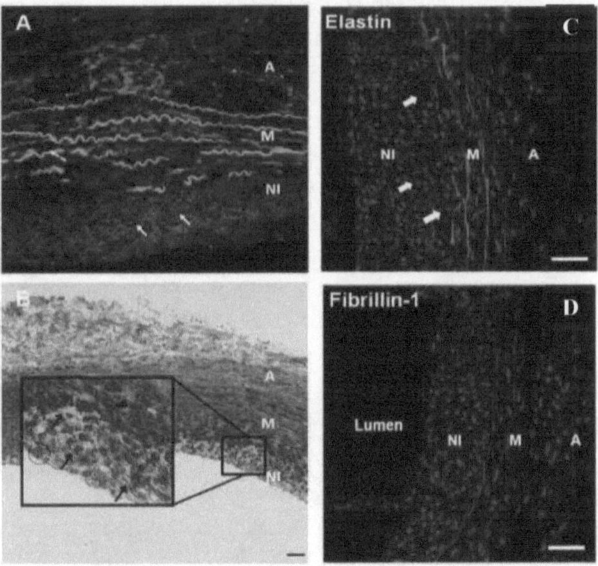

Figure 18: (A) Autofluorescence of elastin in the media and fiber like formation in neo intima. (B) Toluidine blue staining on AAA tissues shows presence of phenotypically different cells in media (elongated) and neointima (epitheloid). (C) Strong fluorescence due to elastin and fibrillin-1 in the media. (D) presence of elastin deposits in the but little fibrillin in the neo intima.

The use of autologous stem cells also provides the advantage of patient-customized treatment while reducing the risk of poor donor compatibility and low chances of complications and infections. Stem cells are readily available from bone marrow, peripheral blood, adipose tissues etc. and have the potential of differentiating into multiple cell types including smooth muscle cells [188]. Hence, these cells can be used as is or by differentiating them into vascular smooth muscle like cells, however, differentiating them into the desired phenotype would be the better option from standpoint of scalability and low incidence and low yield of these cells from source tissues [210]. A different type of stem cells called induced pluripotent stem cells (iPSCs) are recently being studied to improve the scalability. With iPSCs technique, it is possible to generate targeted and individualized cell lines by reprogramming cells from patient's own tissues [211]. However, iPSCs are highly proliferative and therefore carries the risk of tumorigenicity [210]. Progress has been made towards differentiating these cells into desired phenotype and hence subsidize the tumorigenic effect but not fully accomplished. Bone-marrow mesenchymal stem cells (BM-MSCs) would be a potent alternative cell source for elastin regenerative repair because BM-MSCs can readily be differentiated into SMC like cells and have potential anti-inflammatory and immunosuppressive characteristics [212]. Several studies have been performed to demonstrate hypo-immunogenicity of BM-MSCs even upon allogenic transplantation [212]. MSCs have been reported to inhibit T cells and natural killer cells proliferation. MSCs also alters T cell cytokine secretion and cytotoxicity, B-cell maturation and antibody secretion, NK cell cytokine production and cytotoxicity [213]. Both rat and human MSCs express CD90 and MHC class I and MHC class II when activated but they do not express co-stimulatory molecules and therefore do not activate alloreactive T cells. Human MSCs have IL-6, IL-8, IL-12, and TGF-β1 whereas rat MSCs have IL-6, IL-10, IL-12 and TGF-β1. mRNA expression however was found to be greater for anti-inflammatory cytokines than pro-inflammatory [213]. Swaminathan et. al have shown that the secretome of BM-MSCs as well as their smooth muscle like derivative also contain pro-elastogenic and anti-proteolytic cues which imparts matrix regenerative benefits to the resident AAA SMCs while also suppressing the MMP activity [214], [215]. This also shows the possibility of developing cell free approach like delivering BM-SMC secretome components identified to be necessary and sufficient to provide pro-elastogenic and anti-proteolytic benefits using AAA tissue targeting nanoparticles components [216]. **Figure 19** above shows expected role of BM-MSC based cell therapy for AAA repair.

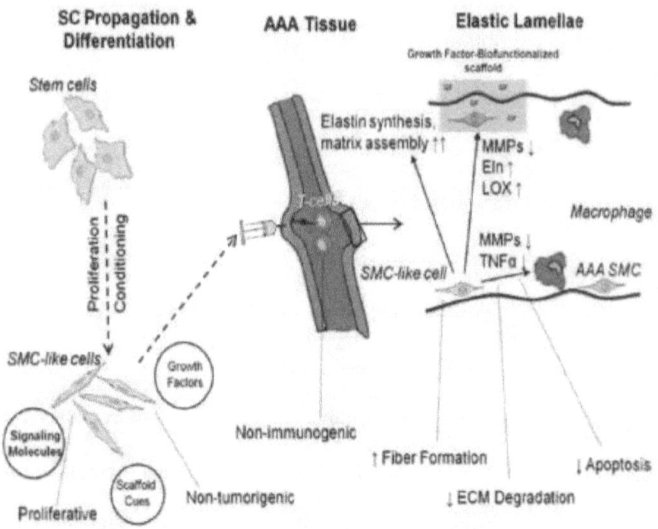

Figure 19: Schematic showing general characteristics and expected role of stem cells in AAA tissue repair and regeneration

The most striking property of BM-MSCs among all stem cells is their natural homing capability to diseased site even though the precise mechanism is yet to be clear. Research shows that homing of BM-MSC is largely dependent on chemokine receptor especially CXCR4 and its ligand stromal derived factor-1 CXCL12 [217]. A study by Wynn et.al has shown the presence of CXCR4 on the subpopulation of MSCs that helps in CXCL12 dependent migration and homing [218]. Similarly, other chemokines involved in MSC migration are CCR1, CCR4, CCR7, CCR10, CCR9, CXCR5 and CXCR6. MSC migration involves a number of steps [217]. It requires the cells to be activated, attached to the endothelial cells, and migrate between the ECs to enter the target. MSCs express a number of adhesion molecules like selectins and integrins which are involved in attachment and migration between the endothelial cells. The binding was shown to be enhanced by activation of ECs with TNF-α. The cells extend podia followed by rolling and adhesion on ECs and migrates. Studies also indicate that binding and rolling of MSCs is mediated by P-selectin molecules and migration is facilitated by binding of VLA-4 present on MSCs with VCAM-1 present on ECs[217]. Therefore, in this body of work we have extensively explored the utility of bone marrow mesenchymal stem cells derived smooth muscle like cells towards elastic matrix regenerative repair in AAAs.

CHAPTER III

**MAINTAINING ELASTOGENICITY OF MESENCHYMAL STEM CELL-
DERIVED SMOOTH MUSCLE CELLS IN 2D CULTURE**

3.1 Introduction

As described in previous chapter, current treatment options for AAAs are surgical but are performed mostly only on large, rupture-prone AAAs bigger than the critical size (maximal diameter > 5.5 cm) and have high procedural risk for many older AAA patients [219]–[221]. Alternative non-surgical treatments to slow, arrest, or even regress small AAAs during their slow (>5 years) growth to rupture is thus mandated.

As mentioned earlier, critical requirement to be able to arrest or regress AAA growth is to restore homeostasis of the structural extracellular matrix (ECM) in the AAA wall. Since, elastic fibers and higher order structures (elastic lamellae) in the aorta wall, which enable vessel stretch and recoil, are unlike collagen in not being able to auto-regenerate or repair post-disruption in adults [212], in the light of chronic matrix breakdown in the AAA wall, it is imperative to provide a major impetus to elastic matrix neoassembly (elastogenesis) concurrent with a deterrent to enzymatic proteolysis, so as to allow for net accumulation of new elastic matrix. Based on literature describing the role of stem cells (SCs) in developmental elastogenesis and vascular tissue repair post-injury [222] as well as previous studies from our lab [6] showing that SMC-like progenitor cells (BM-SMCs) derived from bone marrow mesenchymal stem cells (BM-MSCs) exhibit significantly higher elastogenic capacity than healthy, terminally-differentiated adult vascular SMCs, and are able to stimulate elastic matrix neoassembly by aneurysmal SMCs and in parallel attenuate MMP-mediated elastic matrix breakdown, we subsequently demonstrated that these effects of BM-SMCs in stimulating elastic fiber formation, elastin crosslinking and attenuating MMP activity by aneurysmal SMCs are a) not provided by undifferentiated BM-MSCs[6], and b) mediated by biological factors contained in paracrine secretions (secretome) of the BM-SMCs [6].

SMCs represent a continuum of phenotypic states that span between extreme, but theoretical phenotypes of quiescent, highly contractile and non-synthetic cells ('contractile phenotype') and a highly proliferative, robustly ECM-generating and poorly contractile state ('synthetic phenotype') respectively [223], [224]. While high contractility of terminally differentiated SMCs resident in adult blood vessels allows the vessel to effectively maintain blood pressure, robust ECM synthesis by SMCs in developing vascular tissues and in the injured vascular wall contributes to vascular tissue organization and remodeling/repair respectively [225]. However, most SMCs represent interim phenotypes that can exhibit aspects of both phenotypic extremes [223], [224]. In this context, in prior work [5], we demonstrated that phenotypic co-ordinates of derived BM-SMCs can be altered by modulating conditions of differentiation culture and represent a useful metric to select cells exhibiting superior elastogenicity, contractility, and sufficient proliferative capacity for successful application to regenerative AAA repair. We identified a specific BM-SMC phenotype we now term as cBM-SMCs, that were derived from rat BM-MSCs on a fibronectin (Fn) substrate in the presence of DMEM-F12 medium containing 10% fetal bovine serum (FBS), transforming growth factor –beta (TGF-β1; 2.5 ng/ml) and platelet derived growth factor-ββ (PDGF-ββ; 5 ng/ml) that exhibited superior properties consistent with that listed above. Cell therapy demands large cell inoculates, which in turn necessitates that the differentiated cells be propagated in culture prior to delivery to the collagenous, de-elasticized vascular tissue *in vivo*. Therefore, in this aim we sought to understand how conditions of post-differentiation *in vitro* 2-D culture for the purpose of propagating cBM-SMCs for subsequent *in vivo* use impact their phenotypic, functional, and matrix regenerative properties.

3.2   Materials and Methods

3.2.1   Propagation of rBM-SMCs and cBM-SMCs

Rat bone marrow mesenchymal stem cells (BM-MSCs; Invitrogen, Carlsbad, CA, USA) were differentiated into cBM-SMCs, as described earlier [6]. At 21 days of differentiation the cells were trypsinized and a) seeded on uncoated tissue culture polystyrene flasks and cultured with DMEM F-12 medium containing 10% v/v FBS (Invitrogen) and 1% v/v PenStrep (Thermo Fisher, South Logan, UT) without any growth factors (rBM-SMC) and subsequently passaged upon attaining near-confluence, and b) seeded within human fibronectin- (hFN, 100 ng/ml) coated tissue culture flasks (BD Biosciences, East Rutherford, NJ, USA) cultured with DMEM-F12 medium containing 10% v/v FBS, 1% v/v PenStrep, 2.5 ng/ml of TGF-β1 (Peprotech) and 5 ng/ml of PDGF-BB (Peprotech, Rocky Hill, NJ). These cells, termed cBM-SMCs were subsequently passaged when they attained near confluence and used for further experimentation to compare their phenotypes, and retention of elastogenic and anti-proteolytic effects. In these experiments, healthy rat aortic smooth muscle cells (RASMCs) and BM-MSCs were studied as controls. For transmission electron microscopy (TEM) analysis, EaRASMCs (aneurysmal rat aortic smooth muscle cells) (passage 3-5) (isolated from an elastase injury rat AAA model as we have described previously [5] were cultured as negative controls. The propagation condition of RASMCs (used as positive control) have been previously described [6]. Briefly, the abdominal aorta of three different healthy rats were harvested, cut into small pieces and digested in collagenase type-2 (Worthington Biochemical, Lakewood, NJ) and porcine elastase (Sigma, St. Louis, MO). These digests were then aliquoted equally in each well of six-well plate and cultured in DMEM containing 20% v/v FBS and 1%v/v PenStrep for smooth muscle cell isolation. Once the primary cells adhered and reached confluence, they were passaged and cultured in media containing 10% v/v FBS. Passage 2 RASMCs generated from the 3 different animals were then pooled, passaged, and seeded for culture experiments.

3.2.2   RNA Isolation and Real-Time PCR

The rBM-SMCs were seeded in polystyrene 6-well plate (USA Scientific, Ocala, FL, USA) and cBM-SMCs were seeded in human Fn-coated 6-well plate (BD Biosciences) at 15,000 cells per well (A = 10 cm^2) and cultured for 15 days. Total RNA was isolated from the cultures using a RNeasy mini kit (Qiagen, Valencia, CA, USA) and quantified using a Quant-iT™ Ribogreen® RNA kit (Invitrogen) following manufacturer's instructions. An iScript cDNA synthesis kit (Bio-Rad, Hercules, CA,

USA) was used to synthesize cDNA using 1µg of RNA from all the samples and reverse transcription was performed for total of 40 minutes combining 5 minutes at 25 ˚C, 30 minutes at 42 ˚C and 5 minutes at 85 ˚C according to the manufacturer's instructions. Real time PCR was performed using an Applied Biosystems 7500 Real-Time PCR system with Power SYBR® Green Master Mix (Applied Biosystems). Specially designed primers were used for the 18s (house - keeping gene), α-SMA (*ACTA 2*), caldesmon (*CALD1*), smoothelin (*SMTN*), smooth muscle myosin heavy chain (*MYH11*), Elastin (*ELN*), Fibrillin-1 (*FBN1*), Fibulin-4 (*FBLN4*), Fibulin-5 (*FBLN5*), lysyl oxidase (*LOX*), MMP-2 (*MMP2*), MMP-9 (*MMP9*) and Timp-1 (*TIMP1*). The primers were designed previously in our lab [6], [222], [226]. The PCR data was analyzed using LinReg PCR program. This program uses a MATLAB® code separately for each sample to determine baseline-corrected set of values and window of linearity. PCR efficiency was calculated from the slope of linear fit for each sample. This provided correction for N0. Data value obtained from this analysis was directly used to calculate gene expression ratio as described in literature [227].

3.2.3 Immunofluorescence-Based Detection of SMC Phenotypic Markers and Elastic Matrix Homeostasis Proteins

SMC markers and key proteins involved in elastic fiber hemostasis were detected using immunofluorescence (IF) staining, as described previously [228]. Cells were seeded on coverslips, cultured for 7 days for SMC marker proteins and 21 days for elastin homeostasis proteins, then were fixed using 4% w/v paraformaldehyde for 20 min at 4 °C, permeabilized with 0.1% v/v Triton X-100 (VWR Scientific, West Chester, PA, USA) for 10 min and blocked with PBS containing 5% v/v goat serum

(Gibco Life Technologies, Grand Island, NY). The cells were then incubated overnight with primary antibodies against the SMC marker proteins (Caldesmon, α-SMA, Smoothelin, and myosin heavy chain (MHC)) and elastin homeostasis proteins (Elastin, Fibrillin-1, Fibulin-4, Fibulin-5, LOX, MMP-2, MMP-9 and TIMP-1). The expression of these proteins was then visualized using secondary antibodies conjugated to AlexaFluor 488 or 633 probes (Molecular Probes, Temecula, CA). The coverslips were then mounted on glass slide with Vectashield® mounting medium containing the nuclear dye, 4',6-Diamidine-2'-phenylindole dihydrochloride (DAPI) (Vector Labs, Burlingame, CA). Imaging was done using Olympus I×51 fluorescence microscope (Olympus, Pittsburgh, PA, USA) and the images were analyzed using Image Pro® software.

3.2.4   DNA Assay for Cell Proliferation

DNA content in the cells were quantified using Hoechst Dye based Fluorometric DNA assay protocol developed by Labarca and Paigen [229]. The cell layers at 21 days of culture were harvested in Pi buffer (50mM Na_2HPO_4; 2mM EDTA, and 0.3mM NaN_3) and sonicated to lyse cells and release DNA. The results were quantified assuming 6 pg of DNA contained per cell.

3.2.5   Fastin Assay for Matrix Elastin

At 21 days of culture, the cell layers were harvested in Pi buffer and sonicated. A 0.5-mL aliquot of the sonicated cell layer samples was digested in 0.1 mL of 1.5 M oxalic acid (95 °C, 90 min) and then pelleted by centrifugation at 14,000g. The supernatant containing soluble α-elastin was saved and 0.4 mL of 0.25 M oxalic acid added to the pellet and digested for a further 1 hour at 100 °C. The digestate was centrifuged again and the supernatant pooled with the earlier supernatant fraction. The elastin content in the pooled supernatant was measured using a FASTIN® assay kit (Accurate Chemical and Scientific Corp) as per manufacturer's instructions. The measured elastin content in the samples was normalized to their corresponding DNA content.

3.2.6   Hydroxyproline Assay for Collagen Matrix

A hydroxyproline (OH-Pro) assay was performed to determine the total amount of collagen deposited by the cells in their ECM as described in our published literature [5]. Briefly, the cell layers were harvested in Pi buffer, centrifuged at 2500 rpm for 10 mins and the resulting pellet digested in 1mL of 0.1 M NaOH at 95 °C in a water bath for 1 hour to solubilize elastin and collagen. The digestate was then allowed to cool to room temperature and centrifuged at 2500 rpm. The supernatant containing solubilized collagen was assayed using the OH-Pro assay. Collagen amounts were calculated based on 13.5 % w/w OH-Pro content of collagen.

3.2.7   Estimation of Desmosine Crosslink Content

After 21 days of culture, all four cell types were harvested in phosphate buffered saline (PBS), pH 7.4 and centrifuged for 5 minutes at 500 g to form pellet. The cell pellets were hydrolyzed with 6N HCl for 48 h at 105 °C, evaporated to dryness and reconstituted in 400 µl of water. The samples were then filtered through a 0.45 um filter and desmosine levels determined using a competitive ELISA assay. Total protein in each sample aliquot was measured using ninhydrin assay [230].

3.2.8 Western Blot Analysis

Western blot analysis was performed to semi-quantitatively compare protein expression for the SMC phenotypic marker proteins a-SMA, caldesmon, smoothelin, and MHC, MMPs 2 and 9, tissue inhibitor of matrix metalloprotease -1 (TIMP-1), and lysyl oxidase (LOX), between the four cell types. Briefly, the cells were seeded at a density of 30,000/well in a 6 well plate (n = 6 wells/case) and cultured for 21 days. The cell layers were harvested in RIPA buffer containing a protease inhibitor cocktail (Thermo Scientific, Waltham, MA). The amount of protein in each sample was quantified using BCA assay kit (Thermo Scientific, Waltham, MA). Western blotting was performed as previously described[231]. Briefly, equal volume of protein sample with protein amount within the threshold range of 20 to 30 µg in each cases were taken and mixed with loading buffer. The mixture was reduced and loaded along with a pre-stained molecular weight ladder (Invitrogen) on to 4-12% and 10% SDS-PAGE gels for MW< 60kDa and MW>60kDa proteins respectively. The gels were subjected to dry transfer onto nitrocellulose membranes using iBlot western blotting system (Invitrogen). The membranes were then blocked with Odyssey blocking buffer (LiCOR Biosciences, Lincoln, NE, USA) for 1h at room temperature, and then incubated overnight with respective primary antibodies for different proteins. Following this, the blots were incubated with secondary antibodies against rabbit and mouse conjugated with IRDye® 680LT (1:15000 dilution) and IRDye® 800 CW (1:20000 dilution) respectively. The bands were observed using a LiCOR Odyssey laser-based scanning system, quantified using Image Studio Lite software and quantified as relative density units (RDU) normalized to the intensity the housekeeping protein (β-actin) bands. The advantage of β-actin over other proteins used as loading control (e.g., GADPH) is that it is expressed by all eukaryotic cell types and its expression level does not vary drastically due to cellular treatment or across tissue types [232]. For this reason, it has been adopted as a loading control by many published studies involving assessment of SMCs [233]–[236].

3.2.9   ELISA for MMP-2 and MMP-9 Proteins

Solid Phase ELISA was performed to determine the relative mass values for naturally occurring MMP-2 and MMP-9 using Quantikine® ELISA kit (Catalog # MMP200 and MMP900 respectively; R&D Systems, Minneapolis). Briefly, all four cell types were seeded at 30,000 cells/well in a 6 well plate (n = 6 wells/case). At 21 days of culture they were harvested in RIPA buffer with protease inhibitor cocktail as described above for western blot analysis. The assay reagents and standards were prepared as per manufacturer's instructions. The assay was carried out in 96 well plate adding the appropriate amount of reagents followed by multiple wash steps as indicated in manufacturer's protocol. The optical density was measured using the Cytation 5 plate reader with λ = 450 nm and λ = 570 nm. The absorbance values at 570 nm were subtracted from the values at 450nm to provide corrections for optical imperfections in the plate. Concentration vs optical density graph was plotted for standard curve and log-log plot was used for final calculations.

3.2.10   Transmission Electron Microscopy (TEM)

The ultrastructure of the deposited elastic matrix in all four sets of cultures was visualized using TEM, as we have previously described [237]. Briefly, following 21 days of culture on Permanox® chamber slides (Source) the cell layers were washed with

37 °C PBS, fixed for 5 min at 37 °C followed by overnight fixation with 2.5 w/v glutaraldehyde in 0.1M sodium cacodylate buffer, dehydrated in a graded ethanol series (50-100% v/v), embedded in Epon 812 resin, sectioned, placed on copper grids, stained with uranyl acetate and lead citrate, and visualized on a Hitachi TEM H7600T (High technologies, Pleasanton, CA, USA).

3.2.11 Statistical Analysis

All experiments and analyses were performed on n = 6 replicate cultures per cell type with the following exceptions: [Western blot, n= 3, MMP2 and MMP-9 ELISA, n=3]. Results are reported as mean ± SD with statistical significance of differences determined by one way-ANOVA and deemed for a p value of < 0.05. Sigma Plot 13.0 was used for statistical analysis.

3.3 Results

3.3.1 Gene Expression Profiles of BM-MSCs, RASMCs, and Differentiated SMC types

Results of RT-PCR analysis are presented in **Figure 20**. Gene expression data are shown as log-transformed values of the averages of measured relative fluorescence units (RFUs) since the expression levels differ significantly between genes and cell types, spanning several orders of magnitude. Expression of *ACTA2* was significantly higher in cBM-SMC compared to all other cell types (p < 0.001) whereas *CALD1* expression was significantly higher in the RASMC control (p < 0.001); *CALD1* expression was significantly higher in rBM-SMCs versus cBM-SMCs (p = 0.015).

SMTN expression was not different between the two derived SMC types. *MYH11* expression was the highest among RASMCs and significantly more so than the other cell types (p < 0.001). There were no differences between the two derived phenotypes. *ELN* expression by the cBM-SMCs was significantly higher versus rBM-SMCs (p < 0.001). *ELN* expression by the rBM-SMCs was lower than even BM-MSCs (p = 0.002). Expression of *FBN1*, was significantly higher in both the derived phenotypes compared to RASMCs (p < 0.001) and BM-MSCs (p < 0.05) though there were no differences between them. *FBLN4* expression was significantly higher in cBM-SMC cultures (p = 0.003) than in RASMC cultures and rBM-SMC cultures (p = 0.007) and even more so in BM-MSC cultures. *FBLN4* expression in the BM-MSC cultures was significantly higher than both cBM-SMCs *FBLN5* expression was significantly higher (p<0.05) in cBM-SMC cultures versus RASMCs and BM-MSCs but was not different from the rBM-SMCs. *LOX* expression was significantly higher in cBM-SMC cultures relative all other cell groups (p < 0.001), as also expression of *MMP2* and *MMP9* genes (p < 0.01). TIMP1 expression was similar in all cell types.

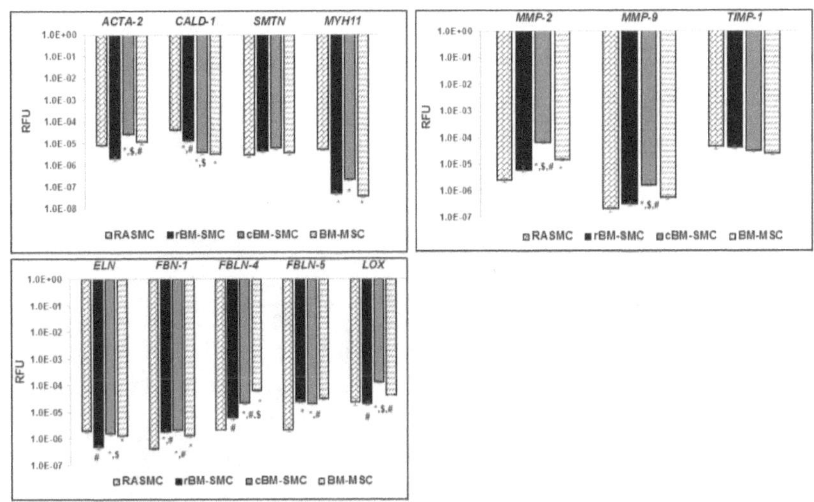

Figure 20: Gene expression profiles for smooth muscle cell marker proteins and elastin homeostasis marker proteins. Cultures of the four different cell types were analyzed using RT-PCR at 15 days of culture. *, \$ and # indicate statistical significance compared to RASMC, cBM-SMC and BM-MSC respectively deemed for p < 0.05

3.3.2 Expression of SMC Phenotypic Marker Proteins and Elastin Homeostasis Proteins

Results of western blot analyses are presented in **Figure 21.** Despite apparent differences expression levels of key SMC marker proteins (Caldesmon, α-SMA, Smoothelin and Myosin Heavy Chain) were not significantly different between the cell groups. Expression of key proteins involved in elastic fiber homeostasis, namely LOX, Fibulin-4, and Fibulin-5 were significantly higher in cBM-SMC cultures than in all other cell groups (p ≤ 0.001, p ≤ 0.005, p ≤ 0.01 respectively). TIMP-1 expression was similar in all groups.

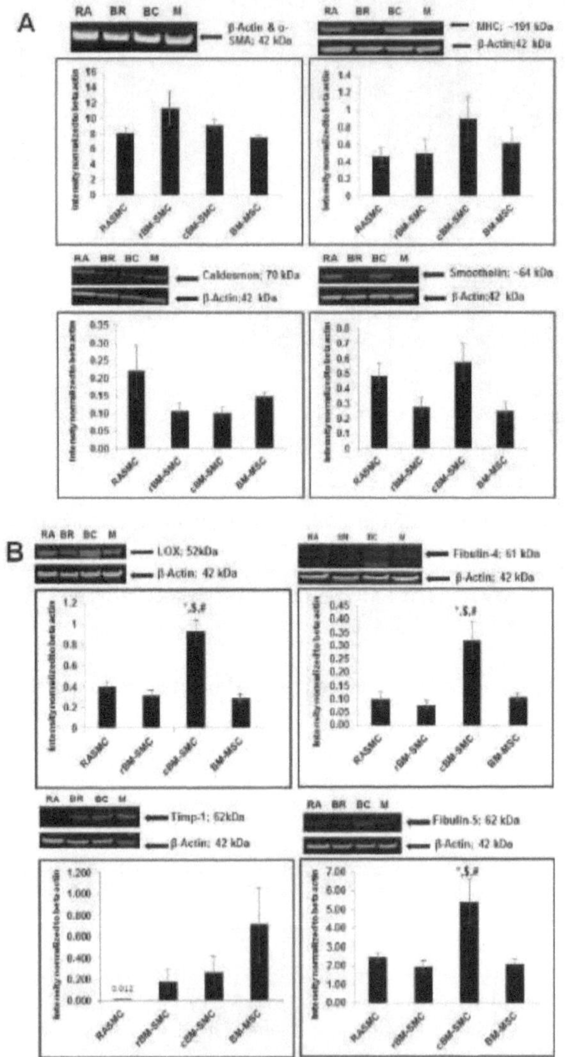

Figure 21: Western blot analysis for expression of SMC marker proteins (A) shows no significance differences between the four cell types. Western blot analysis for expression of key elastic matrix assembly proteins (B) indicates significantly higher LOX, Fibulin-4 and Fibulin-5 expression by cBM-SMCs whereas no significant differences were found among the four cell types in TIMP-1 expression. *, $ and # indicate statistical significance compared to RASMC, cBM-SMC and BM-MSC respectively deemed for p < 0.05. The blots are brightness/contrast enhanced however the values represent analysis performed on unsaturated bands. RA, BR, BC and M in the blot represents RASMCs, rBM-SMCs, cBM-SMCs and BM-MSCs respectively

73

As shown in **Figure 22**, total MMP-2 protein synthesis was significantly higher in cBM-SMC cultures compared to RASMCs (p < insert value), rBM-SMC (p < 0.001) and BM-MSC (p = 0.006) Expression of the active MMP-2 isoform was again the highest in cBM-SMC cultures (p < 0.001 vs. other groups), followed by the rBM-SMCs (p = 0.002 vs. RASMC and p = 0.039 vs. BM-MSCs). Expression ratios of active MMP-2 to TIMP-1 were significantly higher in cBM-SMC cultures than in RASMC cultures (p = 0.03) but were found to be not different versus rBM-SMCs and BM-MSCs. MMP9 was not detected on the western blots. The results of IF (**Figure 23**) also qualitatively represents and validates the amount of expression of these SMC markers and elastin homeostasis proteins.

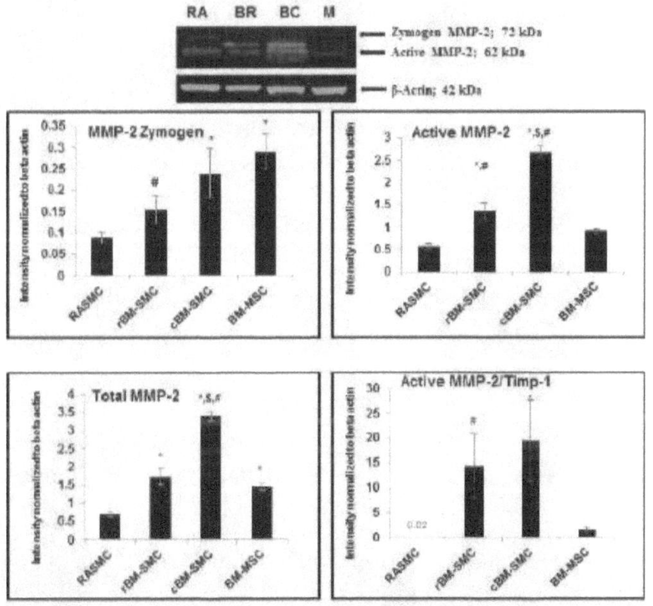

Figure 22: Western blot analysis for MMP-2 protein expression. The figure compares expression of MMP-2 zymogen, active MMP-2, and total MMP-2 by all four cell types as also measures of net proteolytic activity, i.e., ratios of active MMP-2 to TIMP-1. *, $ and # indicate statistical significance compared to RASMC, cBM-SMC and BM-MSC respectively deemed for p < 0.05. RA, BR, BC and M in the blot represents RASMCs, rBM-SMCs, cBM-SMCs and BM-MSCs respectively

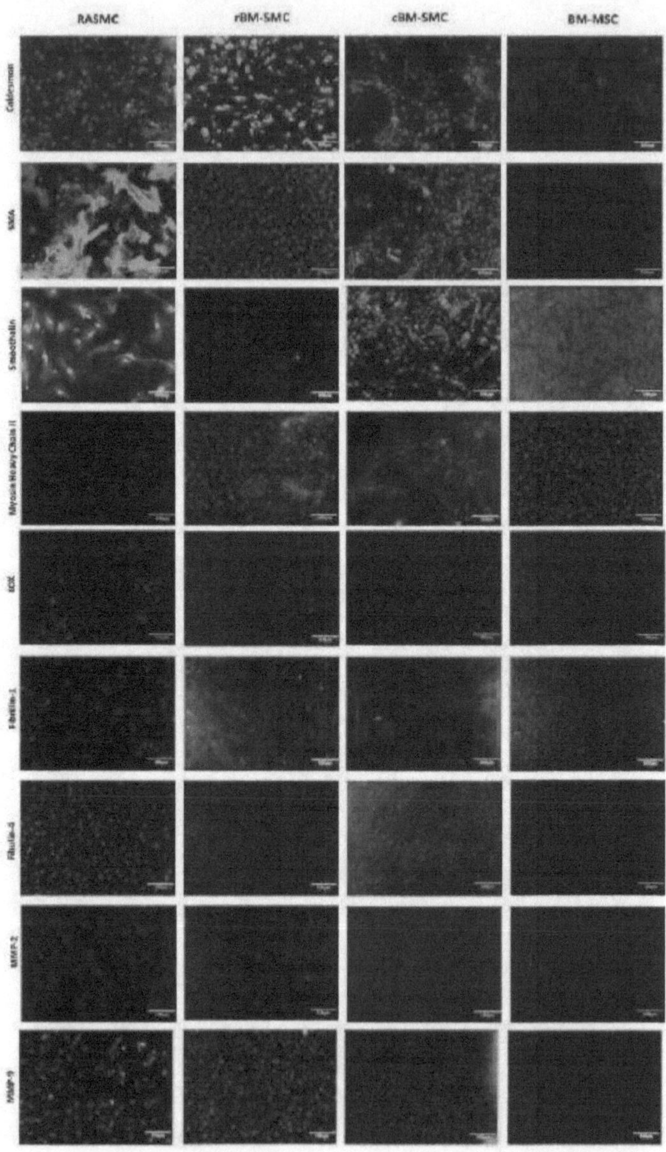

Figure 23: Comparative expression of SMC marker proteins and key elastic fiber assembly proteins by derived and control cell types using immunofluorescence. Expression trends conform to that deemed by western blot analysis

3.3.3 Cell Proliferation

A DNA assay showed increase in DNA content (i.e., number of cells) over 21 days to be significantly lower in the derived cell types (and RASMCs) relative to BM-MSCs ($p < 0.001$) and significantly higher versus RASMCs ($p < 0.001$) (**Figure 24A**). There were no differences in cell proliferation between the rBM-SMCs and c-BM-SMCs.

3.3.4 Elastic Matrix Synthesis

Figures 24B and C show elastic matrix amounts deposited in cell cultures on an absolute and cell number-normalized basis respectively. Total matrix elastic matrix protein amounts were significantly higher in both the derived phenotypes compared to RASMC ($p < 0.001$) but lower compared to BM-MSCs ($p < 0.004$). However, on a cell normalized basis elastic matrix production by the RASMCs was significantly higher than by the cBM-SMCs, rBM-SMCs and BM-MSCs ($p < 0.001$). There were no differences in elastic matrix synthesis on a per cell basis between cBM-SMCs and rBM-SMCs.

3.3.5 Desmosine Crosslink Content

As indicated in **Figure 24D**, on a protein content normalized basis, desmosine crosslink content in cBM-SMC cultures was significantly higher than in other cases ($p < 0.003$).

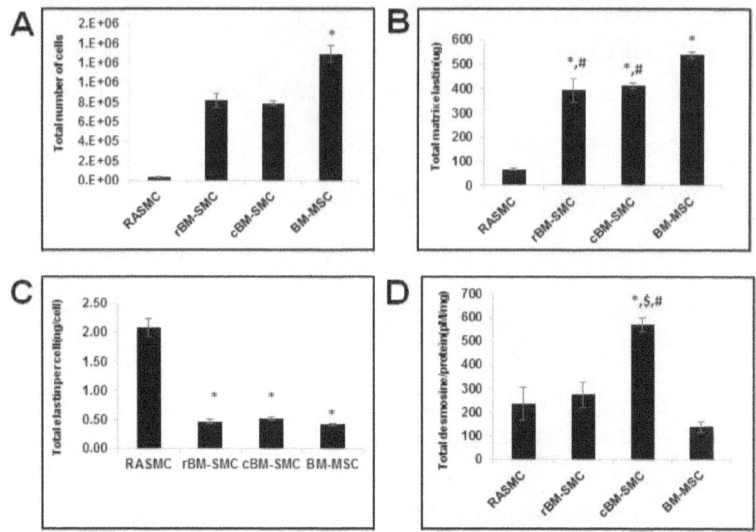

Figure 24: Differences between derived SMC subtypes and RASMC and BM-MSC controls in cell proliferation (A), elastic matrix production on a total (B) and per cell (C) basis and desmosine crosslinking of the matrix (D). In all cases, 30,000 cells were seeded per well in a 6-well plate and cultured for 21 days before analysis. *, $ and # indicate statistical significance compared to RASMC, cBM-SMC and BM-MSC respectively deemed for p < 0.05

3.3.6   Collagen Matrix Deposition

Results of a hydroxyproline assay (**Figure 25**) indicated little collagen matrix in RASMC cultures and significantly higher amounts in all other tested cell types ($p \leq$ 0.001); there were no significant differences in collagen synthesis between the two derived SMC subtypes and between these cultures and BM-MSC cultures. On a per cell normalized basis, collagen content was again higher in the differentiated SMC cultures compared to RASMCs ($p < 0.001$) and BM-MSCs ($p < 0.02$) but not different between the cBM-SMCs and rBM-SMCs. BM-MSC also had significantly higher collagen/cell compared to RASMC ($p = 0.01$).

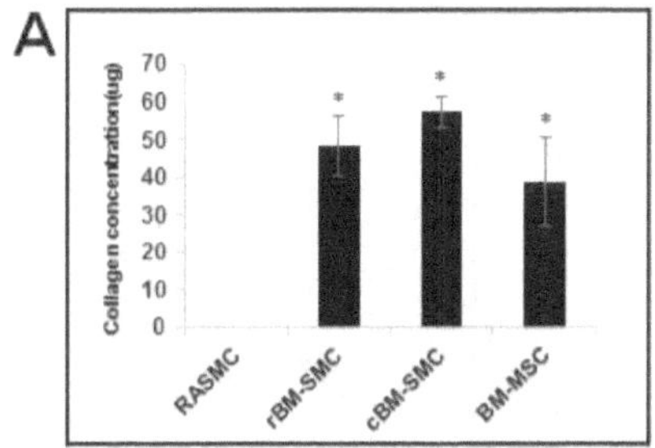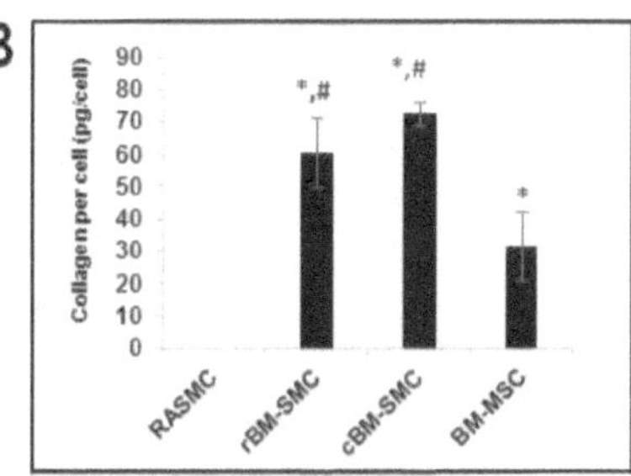

Figure 25: Cell-type specific differences in collagen synthesis measured using a hydroxyproline assay shown in absolute amounts (A) and amounts on a cell-normalized basis (B). No significant differences were found between the two derived cell types however cell normalized collagen content was higher in both of them compared to RASMC and BM-MSC. * and # indicate statistical significance compared to RASMC and BM-MSC respectively deemed for p < 0.05

3.3.7 MMP-2 and MMP-9 Protein Synthesis

Synthesis of MMP-2 (72 kDa, 66 kDa isoforms) and MMP-9 (82 kDa, 72 kDa isoforms) proteins were measured using ELISA and results are shown in **Figure 26**. MMP-2 protein synthesis was significantly higher in cBM-SMC cultures compared to all other cell types ($p \leq 0.003$) which is consistent with western blot results. rBM-SMC also generated significantly higher amounts of MMP-2 protein compared to RASMC ($p = 0.002$) and BM-MSC ($p = 0.038$), but less so than did the cBM-SMCs ($p = 0.003$). MMP-9 protein was not expressed in RASMC and cBM-SMC cultures. MMP-9 synthesis by rBM-SMCs was significantly higher ($p \leq 0.005$) compared to all other cell types.

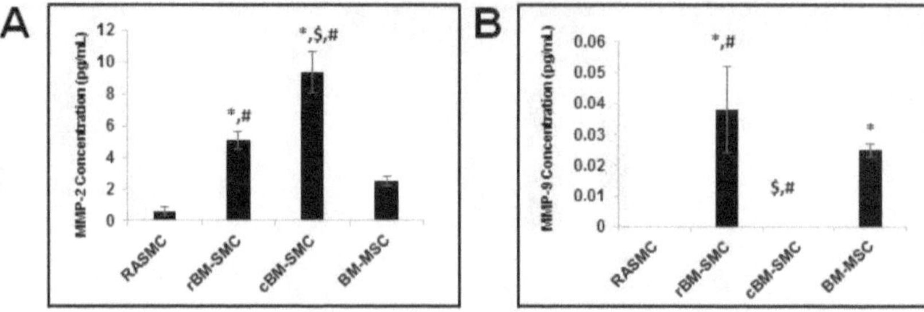

Figure 26: Protein concentrations of MMP-2 (A) and MMP-9 (B) measured in cell layers, measured using ELISA. Results show significantly higher MMP-2 protein amounts in cBM-SMC cultures compared to rBM-SMC, RASMC, and BM-MSC cultures, and significantly lower MMP-9 protein amounts relative to rBM-SMC and BM-MSC cultures. *, \$ and # indicate statistical significance compared to RASMC, cBM-SMC and BM-MSC respectively deemed for p < 0.05

3.3.8   Elastic Matrix Ultrastructure

TEM (**Figure 27**) showed presence of a homogenously dense matrix composed of forming elastic fibers in the cBM-SMC cultures, and noticeably less dense elastic matrix deposition in the rBM-SMC cultures. The forming fibers were comprised of both essential components, namely the microfibrillar pre-scaffold (white arrows) on to which crosslinked amorphous elastin coacervates (red arrows) were deposited. In contrast, elastic fiber deposition was poor in RASMC and EaRASMC cultures and only sporadic, amorphous elastin clumps were seen.

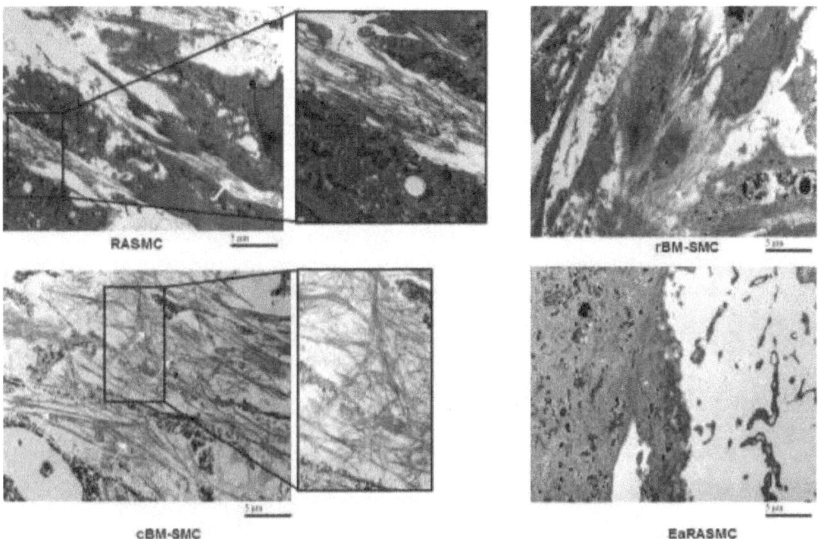

Figure 27: Transmission electron micrographs showing significantly greater density of forming elastic fibers (red arrows) in cBM-SMC cultures, and less so in rBM-SMC cultures relative to RASMC cultures, which contained mainly amorphous elastin deposits (white arrows). Very few amorphous elastin deposits and no fibers were seen in EaRASMC cultures

3.4 Discussion

In this aim, we have sought to determine if continued provision of differentiation conditions (fibronectin substrate, TGF-β and PDGF-BB) is essential to maintain the phenotype and matrix synthesis properties of BM-SMCs during their propagation in 2D culture, prior to delivery *in vivo*. To confirm differentiation of BM-MSCs into SMCs, we investigated the expression of SMC phenotypic markers by our generated BM-SMC culture groups. While SMA is expressed by the SMCs even early in their differentiation, caldesmon is expressed in the mid stage of differentiation. On the other hand, smoothelin and myosin heavy chain is a marker that is exclusively expressed by contractile SMCs[225]. The RT-PCR results showed the derived cells to be similar to healthy RASMCs in exhibiting contractile SMC markers, but to not be terminally differentiated. The cBM-SMCs robustly expressed *ACTA2* but not *MYH11* suggesting that they are not terminally differentiated as are the RASMCs and SMCs in native vessels but are rather of an early or intermediate SMC phenotype. *SMTN* and *MYH11* expression being similar between the two derived cell types, higher *CALD1* expression by the BM-SMCs points to their relatively higher maturation vs the cBM-SMCs. Despite the differences in gene expression profiles, expression of SMC marker proteins was not statistically different between the cell groups, quite possibly due to the western blot analysis being less precise and data hence generating with relatively large variability. Regardless, this western blot data confirms our derived cell types to be SMC-like. The limited expression of these same SMC markers by the undifferentiated BM-MSCs on the other hand has been described in literature [238].

Superior elastogenic properties are critical to selection of cells towards application to AAA wall repair. One of the major players in regulation of elastin homeostasis and vessel remodeling is lysyl oxidase (LOX), a copper dependent amine oxidase which enables elastin crosslinking and consequent stabilization. LOX downregulation is thought to have central role in instability of plaque leading to destructive remodeling like it takes place in case of aneurysm [239]. We found significantly higher *LOX* gene expression and protein synthesis in cBM-SMC cultures than in all other cell groups suggesting a better crosslinked and proteolysis-resistant elastic matrix in those cultures. This may be due to the continued presence of TGF-β1 which is known to upregulate both LOX gene expression and protein synthesis [240]. Fibronectin in the cell substrate, is also known to bind LOX and LOXL1 proenzymes, and also activate BMP-1 and through the auspices of the latter, proteolytically cleave the proenzymes to release active LOX enzyme [241], [242], increasing LOX activity. Another important measure of elastin crosslinking is desmosine which is a tetra - functional amino acid that links elastin molecules. Desmosine content was significantly higher in the cBM-SMC cultures than in the other culture groups, likely as a result of higher LOX synthesis/activity. In addition, fibronectin facilitates deposition of the fibrillin-1 micro fibrils [243], [244] which are a pre-requisite to initiate elastic matrix / fiber assembly which is consistent with increased elastic matrix fiber deposition in cBM-SMCs cultures. More specifically, fibrillin-1 is deposited as a pre-scaffold upon which elastin is deposited and coacervates and extends to form a matrix fiber [245], [246]. Fibrillin-1 expression by cBM-SMCs is likely increased in presence of exogenous TGF-β [247].

Fibulins 4 and 5 coacervate tropoelastin to facilitate their integration with fibrillin-1 microfibrils for crosslinking by either LOX (Fibulin-4) [248] or its homologue LOXL1 (Fibulin-5) [249], [250] to which they also bind to promote elastic fiber assembly. In fact, a mutation in the homozygous fibulin-4, has been implicated in AAA pathophysiology [251]. In our study, gene expression and protein synthesis of both fibulins-4 and 5 was the highest in cBM-SMC cultures, followed by in the rBM-SMC cultures. While fibulin-4 facilitates LOX binding to both fibrillin-1 and tropoelastin nuclei and processes it to an enzymatically active form [248], fibulin-5 similarly regulates the LOX isoform, LOXL1, expressed typically in adult cells [252]. The higher expression of fibulins-4 and -5 in cBM-SMC cultures thus implies improved elastic matrix deposition and fiber formation which was the case. In this context, our study outcomes were also consistent with our earlier data in showing that elastin expression by cBM-SMCs is significantly higher than expression by BM-MSCs and

RASMCs [6]. On the other hand, elastic matrix synthesis by rBM-SMCs was below levels in BM-MSC cultures, which may be related to the absence of any supplemented growth factors, though further investigation is warranted. However, no differences in elastic matric deposition were noted on a per cell basis between the derived SMC types, which were higher than in BM-MSC cultures, and in the case of cBM-SMCs, similar to the RASMCs. This discrepancy between the PCR data and Fastin assay data can be attributed to the fact that elastic matrix assembly not only depends on post-transcriptional processes resulting in synthesis of elastin precursors, but also a complex hierarchical process of fiber assembly involving parallel or sequential involvement of numerous other elastic fiber assembly proteins (LOX, Fibulins, Fibrillins, Fibronectin), several of which were upregulated in cBM-SMC cultures versus the other cell types. In addition, total elastic matrix amounts generated by cBM-SMCs are significantly greater than RASMCs due to their more rapid proliferation post-seeding. Since, the benefits of a matrix regenerative cell therapy, as we propose, ultimately depends upon total amount of new elastic matrix generated, both our derived SMC types may be deemed superior to the RASMCs, although greater expression of elastic fiber homeostasis proteins by the cBM-SMCs point to their likely superior elastogenic properties versus rBM-SMCs. Supporting these results, TEM **(Figure 27)** showed robust deposition of a fibrous elastic matrix (white arrows) in the extracellular space within cBM-SMC cultures, less so in rBM-SMC cultures, and only sporadic deposition of fibrous elastin and amorphous elastin clumps (red arrows) in RASMC and EaRASMC cultures. Our data in **Figures 21-26** also suggest that elastic fiber formation by BM-MSCs is also likely to be poor due to the much lower expression of the key proteins involved in elastic fiber assembly proteins though total elastic matrix deposition itself is high due to high proliferative capacity of these cells. This, in addition to the lack of pro-elastogenic effects of the undifferentiated BM-MSCs on aneurysmal SMCs [5], [6], which we determined in an early study render them less efficacious for cell therapy aimed at regenerating elastic matrix.

While our data collectively suggest that phenotype influences elastic matrix assembly properties of BM-MSC-derived SMCs, no differences were noted in collagen matrix deposition between the cBM-SMCs and rBM-SMCs, which were significantly higher than that in RASMC cultures. In the latter, collagen amounts were below the limit of detection, which can be at least in part attributed to low cell numbers owing to the intrinsically poor proliferative capacity of RASMCs. While MMP-2 protein synthesis measured by western blot and ELISA was higher in cBM-SMC cultures, MMP-9 was not, consistent with gene expression trends. The findings as to low expression of MMP-9 are also consistent with prior observations by our group [5], [6], [167]. This may be owed to poor constitutive expression of MMP-9 by SMCs in culture, which is well documented [253]. Since MMP-2 and MMP-9 are countered by TIMP-1, MMP-2/TIMP-1 ratios protein ratios were compared between the culture groups. The MMP-2/TIMP-1 ratios observed in the cBM-SMC cultures was higher versus the RASMCs which might be considered a sub-optimal outcome. This could be possibly attributed to the pro-MMP-2 effects of the TGF-β at certain doses [254] specially in the absence of it is sequestration in the absence of a 3-D ECM. Regardless, cBM-SMCs can be deemed the superior derived phenotype owing to their lack of MMP-9 expression, unlike the rBM-SMCs.

Therefore, this chapter shows that propagation of the differentiated BM-SMCs *in vitro* 2-D culture must necessarily be performed in the continued presence of differentiation culture conditions in order to maintain their phenotype. The results have vital implications to successful generation of large cBM-SMC populations for subsequent use in cell therapy for AAAs. In next chapter we have separately demonstrated that our differentiated cBM-SMCs maintain the pro-elastogenic and anti-proteolytic benefits when introduced into a de-elasticized collagen-rich tissue milieu and thereafter maintained in the absence of differentiation growth factors or Fn.

CHAPTER IV

**PRO-ELASTOGENIC EFFECTS OF MESENCHYMAL STEM CELL
DERIVED SMOOTH MUSCLE CELLS IN A 3D COLLAGENOUS MILIEU**

4.1 Introduction

Intrinsically poor auto-regenerative repair of proteolytically-disrupted elastic matrix structures by resident SMCs in the wall of abdominal aortic aneurysms (AAAs) prevents growth arrest and regression of these wall expansions. While loss of collagen in AAAs is compensated by exuberant synthesis of new collagen fibers [255], elastic fibers, which impart tissue stretch and recoil properties, do not naturally regenerate or repair [256], due to deficient and impaired elastogenesis by adult and diseased vascular smooth muscle cells (SMCs) [1] as stated earlier. Due to this, restoring AAA wall structure to a healthy state has not been possible. Cell therapy can potentially address this problem by providing an elastogenic stimulus to aneurysmal SMCs, compensating for apoptotic cell death in the AAA wall, serving as a robust new source of new elastic matrix, and providing a deterring proteolysis in the AAA wall.

In earlier aim [257], we identified a non-terminally differentiated phenotype of SMC-like cells (cBM-SMCs) derived from rat bone marrow mesenchymal stem cells

(BM-MSCs) which exhibit superior elastogenicity relative to even healthy rat aortic SMCs and which uniquely provide paracrine pro-elastogenic and anti-proteolytic stimuli to aneurysmal SMCs in culture. These cells were differentiated in 2-dimensional (2D), fibronectin-coated substrates in the presence of exogenous Transforming Growth Factor- β1 (TGF-β1) and Platelet Derived Growth Factor-BB (PDGF-ββ). We demonstrated that these cells maintain their differentiated phenotype and maintain their beneficial pro-matrix regenerative/anti-proteolytic properties when propagated long term under the same culture conditions. In this aim we sought to determine how elastic matrix neo-assembly by the cBM-SMCs is modulated by a 3-D collagenous, tissue milieu evocative of the AAA wall tissue to which these cells will be delivered for therapy. Since it is difficult to delineate matrix neo-assembly from gross changes to elastin homeostasis *in vivo*, we will investigate this aspect in a cell-compacted collagen gel culture model, wherein previous studies suggest that SMCs seeded within collagen gels actively remodel in a manner similar to that in the medial layer of the aorta [258]. The 3-D collagenous milieu is also known to promote contractile phenotype of SMCs which is not conducive to elastin synthesis [259], and hence represents a more rigorous system to compare elastogenicity of cBM-SMCs to undifferentiated BM-MSCs and healthy rat aortic SMCs (RASMCs) in standalone cultures, and assess their pro-elastogenic and anti-proteolytic effects on rat aneurysmal SMCs in co-cultures. Therefore, in this aim, we further investigated the ability of the cBM-SMCs to maintain the superior elastogenic properties in a 3D collagenous milieu alone and in co-culture with EaRASMC to evaluate their potential as an alternative cell source for cell therapy in AAA.

4.2 Materials and Methods

4.2.1 Generation of healthy and aneurysmal SMCs

All animal procedures were conducted with approval of the Institutional Animal Care and Use Committee (IACUC) at the Cleveland Clinic. Healthy rat aortic smooth muscle cells (RASMCs) were isolated from rat aortal segments harvested from multiple healthy male Sprague-Dawley rats (120-150g) and aneurysmal rat aortic smooth muscle cells (EaRASMCs) were isolated from rats induced with AAAs via elastase infusion-mediated aortal injury as we have earlier published [166]. The cells were isolated from the harvested aortal tissues from 3 separate animals as per our published explant culture technique [167] and pooled prior to propagation and passaging (<P6) prior to use. Briefly, healthy and AAA containing aortal segments were cut open longitudinally and the intima layer scraped off gently with a scalpel. The medial layer was separated from the underlying adventitial layer and cut into ~0.5 mm long slices and washed twice with warm, sterile phosphate-buffered saline (PBS). The tissue slices were enzymatically digested with Dulbecco's Modified Eagle Medium (DMEM/F12) (Invitrogen, Carlsbad, CA, USA) containing 125 U/mg of collagenase (Worthington Biochemicals, Lakewood, NJ, USA) and 3 U/mg of elastase (Worthington Biochemicals) for 30 minutes at 37 °C, centrifuged (400g, 5 minutes) and cultured for over 2 weeks in T-75 flasks. The cells were cultured in DMEM/F12 medium supplemented with 10% v/v fetal bovine serum (FBS; PAA Laboratories, Etobicoke, Ontario, Canada) and 1% v/v penicillin–streptomycin (Penstrep; Thermo-Fisher, South Logan, UT, USA). The primary EaRASMCs and RASMCs obtained from these tissue explants were propagated for a further 2 weeks and were used for experiments until passage 5.

4.2.2 Directed differentiation of BM-MSCs into cBM-SMCs

For propagation, the BM-MSCs of three different rat cell lines were pooled and then seeded onto T-25 tissue culture polystyrene flasks (USA Scientific, Ocala, FL, USA) at a density of 2×10^3 cells/cm^2 and cultured in low-glucose DMEM medium (Invitrogen), supplemented with 10% v/v MSC-qualified FBS (Invitrogen, Carlsbad, CA, USA) and 1% v/v pen-strep (Thermo-Fisher, Waltham, MA). When the cell layer was confluent, the cells were trypsinized and re-were seeded in human fibronectin (hFN, 100 ng/ml)-coated tissue culture flasks (BD Biosciences, East Rutherford, NJ, USA). The cells were cultured in serum-free Multipotent Adult Progenitor Cell (MAPC) differentiation medium at a density of 2×10^3 per cm^2 in a human fibronectin (hFn) coated flask for 6 days as described before. In the subsequent 5 days, the cells were cultured in medium containing 2% v/v FBS, 2.5 ng/ml of TGF-β (Peprotech, Rocky Hill, NJ, USA) and 5 ng/ml of PDGF-$\beta\beta$ (R&D Systems, Minneapolis, MN, USA). The transformation of the cells from cobblestone to elongated morphology, indicated successful differentiation. Successful differentiation of the BM-MSCs into the desired SMC phenotype was confirmed by western blot and immunofluorescence (IF) analysis for key SMC marker proteins as performed as we have earlier published [5]. The cells were then passaged and propagated further for 10 days under the same culture conditions. At this point the cells are considered as passage 0 (P0) BM-SMCs. Cells from 3 different animals were pooled and used in experiments at passages <5.

4.2.3 Preparing cell-compacted collagen constructs

Cell-compacted collagen gel constructs were fabricated as we have earlier published [259]. Briefly, acid solubilized type-I collagen (Gibco™, ThermoFisher Scientific) was mixed with 5× DMEM F-12 medium and neutralized with 0.1 N NaOH to pH 7.0. BM-SMCs, RASMCs, and BM-MSCs, either alone or as 1:1 number ratio of these cells with EaRASMCs were mixed with the pH-neutralized collagen solution to generate a mixture containing 2 mg/ml of collagen, and 1×10^6 cells/ ml of mixture (constructs analyzed by histology) or 5×10^5 cells/ml (constructs subject to biochemical analysis) and 20% v/v FBS. Higher cell density was used for histology to make elastin more prominent for visualization. A 2mL volume of this cell suspension was aliquoted around a cloning ring (Sigma-Aldrich®, St.Louis, MO, USA) centrally placed within the wells of a 12-well plate. After gelation around the cloning rings, the constructs were allowed to compact around the cloning rings, due to the contractility of the embedded cells while cultured in medium containing 10% v/v FBS for 21 days and then assayed.

4.2.4 Assessing contractility of cell-seeded constructs

The constructs were imaged in a non-fluorescence photographic mode on an IVIS Spectrum CT (PerkinElmer, Waltham, MA, USA) and the progressive contraction of gels was measured using the Image J® software at different time points over 21 days of culture. Briefly, at day 0, the area occupied by the gelled constructs for all the cases were same which was calculated as,

$$Gel\ area = Well\ area - Cloning\ ring\ area$$

At the subsequent time points. The area was calculated as,

$$Gel\ area = Total\ area - Cloning\ ring\ area$$

wherein the Total area refers to the area occupied by the contracted construct including the cloning ring.

4.2.5 Estimating cellularity within constructs

The proliferation of cells within the collagen gels was estimated using a fluorometric DNA assay as previously published [260]. Briefly, after 21 days in culture, the collagen constructs were flash-frozen in liquid nitrogen, lyophilized and their dry tissue weights measured. The samples were then digested in 10 mg/ml of proteinase-K (Invitrogen, Carlsbad, CA, USA; 65 °C, 10 hours) and subsequently boiled (100 °C, 10 minutes) to neutralize enzyme activity [261]. The solubilized samples were diluted in Pi buffer (50 mM of Na_2HPO_4, 2 mM of EDTA and 0.3 mM of NaN_3), pH 7.4, sonicated, and the DNA content measured using the fluorometric Hoechst 33258 dye-based assay described by Labarca & Paigen[10]. Cell numbers were estimated assuming 6 pg of DNA/cell. The results were represented as cell number normalized to the dry weight of the construct.

4.2.6 Quantifying elastic matrix content within constructs

At 21 days of culture, the compacted collagen constructs were lyophilized, and their dry weights measured. They were then digested in 1 ml of 0.1 N NaOH (98 °C, 1 hour) to convert alkali-soluble matrix elastin into the α-elastin form. The samples were then centrifuged (1456g, 10 minutes) and the supernatant fraction (first fraction of elastin, designated S1) collected for analysis of alkali-soluble elastin content. The pelleted fractions (P1) were re-suspended in 0.25 M of oxalic acid and digested (98°C, 1 hour) to convert alkali-insoluble matrix elastin into the α-elastin form. After digestion, the fractions were filter-centrifuged (13,000rpm, 10 minutes) with 10 kDa cut-off membranes (Millipore). The solubilized matrix elastin retained above the filters were reconstituted. Both the elastin fractions (S1, P1) were assayed using a FASTIN® assay kit (Accurate Chemical and Scientific Corp, Westbury, NY) as per the manufacturer's instructions. The results were normalized to the dry weight of the constructs.

4.2.7   Estimating desmosine crosslinks within the constructs

At 21 days of culture, the cell-compacted collagen constructs were rinsed in (PBS) and pelleted by centrifugation (5824g, 10 minutes). The supernatant was discarded, and the pellet lyophilized, then hydrolyzed with 6N HCl (105 °C, 48 hours), evaporated to dryness in a stream of nitrogen and reconstituted in 400 µl of water. These samples were then filtered through a 0.45-µm Amicon filter (Sigma Aldrich) and desmosine levels determined using a competitive ELISA assay [6]. Total protein in each sample aliquot was measured using the ninhydrin assay [230].

4.2.8   Morphometric analysis of elastin in histological sections and fluorescence-detection of elastin

Morphometric analysis of elastic fibers present in the extracellular matrix of each group of constructs was performed on Image Pro Plus® (Media Cybernetics, Inc. Rockville, Maryland, USA). Briefly, at 21 days of culture, the collagen constructs were fixed overnight in 4% v/v PFA (Electron Microscopy Sciences, Hatfield, PA, USA). The constructs were paraffin embedded and then sectioned (8 microns thickness) and stained with Verhoeff-Van Gieson stain which stains elastin fibers in purple to black color. The whole stained slides were scanned at 20x magnification using a Leica

SCN400F slide scanner (Leica Microsystems, Wetzlar, Germany) and the images were exported as SCN files for viewing and subsequent conversion to .tiff format. The images were then imported into Image Pro® and whole sections were selected as the region of interest (ROI) for analysis. The pixels corresponding to the VVG stained structures were manually selected within the ROI and an inbuilt macro was used to quantify percent area and minimum diameter of the fibers. The values were exported to excel for further analysis.

To visualize the autofluorescence of elastin, the paraffin embedded slides were treated with xylene 2X for 5 minutes each and dehydrated with 95% ethanol for 5 minutes. The sections were then treated with 0.05% w/v Pontamine Sky Blue (MP Biomedicals, Solon, OH) for 30 mins and mounted with Vectashield mounting medium, cover-slipped and observed with a visible red fluorescent filter in Leica TCS-SP8-AOBS inverted confocal microscope (Leica Microsystems, Wetzlar, Germany). Pontamine Sky Blue transfers the autofluorescence of elastin alone to the red region of the spectrum in addition to quenching the autofluorescence of both elastin and collagen [262].

4.2.9 Western blot for MMP-2 and MMP-9

Synthesis of MMP-2 and MMP-9 proteins in the collagen constructs seeded with single cell types were semi-quantitatively compared with western blots. At 21 days of culture, the cell-compacted constructs were harvested, extracted in RIPA buffer with 1% w/v protease inhibitor cocktail (Thermo-Scientific) and sonicated (4 °C, 1 min). For each set of constructs, equal volumes of the extracted proteins containing 20-30 µg of protein were mixed with loading buffer. The mixture was reduced and loaded along with a pre-stained molecular weight ladder (Invitrogen, Carlsbad, CA, USA) on to 10%

SDS-PAGE gels (Invitrogen, Carlsbad, CA, USA). The gels were dry transferred onto

nitrocellulose membranes using iBlot® western blotting system (Invitrogen). The

membranes were then blocked with Odyssey blocking buffer (LiCOR Biosciences,

Lincoln, NE, USA) (1hour room temperature) and then incubated overnight with

primary antibodies against MMP-2 (Abcam, Cambridge, UK), MMP-9 (Abcam,

Cambridge, UK) and β-actin (Sigma Aldrich). Following this, the blots were incubated

with secondary antibodies against rabbit and mouse conjugated with IRDye® 680LT

(1:15000 v/v) and IRDye® 800 CW (1:20000 v/v) (LiCOR Biosciences) respectively.

The bands were observed using a LiCOR Odyssey laser-based scanning system,

quantified using Image Studio Lite® Software (LiCOR Biosciences) and quantified as

relative density units (RDU) normalized to the intensity of the loading control (β-actin)

bands. β-actin was selected as loading control because it is expressed by all the

eukaryotic cells and its expression level does not alter drastically due to cellular

treatment across tissue types [233]·[234]·[263]·[236].

4.2.10 Statistical Analysis

All the statistical analysis was performed in Sigma Plot 13.0 software. The

results are presented in box plot (except for contractility which is presented as mean

±SD) showing mean, median, 10th, 25th, 75th and 90th percentile and each individual

values are represented by colored dots. n=6 cells seeded constructs were used for all

the biochemical analysis and n=3 cell seeded constructs were used for histological

assessments. All the comparisons were performed using One Way Analysis of Variance

(ANOVA) with Fisher LSD method for multiple comparisons. $p < = 0.05$ were considered statistically significant.

4.3   Results

4.3.1   Contraction of cellularized constructs

Results comparing contraction of the different groups of cellularized collagen constructs are shown in **Figure 28**. Collagen constructs seeded with cBM-SMCs alone contracted to a significantly higher degree relative to constructs seeded with RASMCs alone and BM-MSCs alone. Similarly, contraction of constructs was significantly higher in cocultures of cBM-SMCs with EaRASMCs versus constructs seeded with EaRASMCs alone, and with RASMCs and EaRASMCs together.

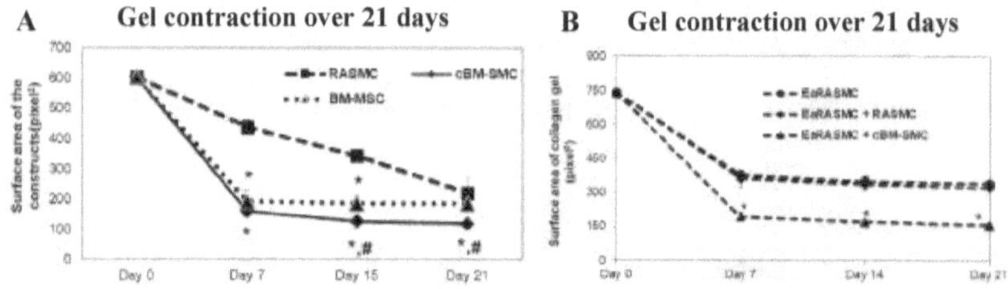

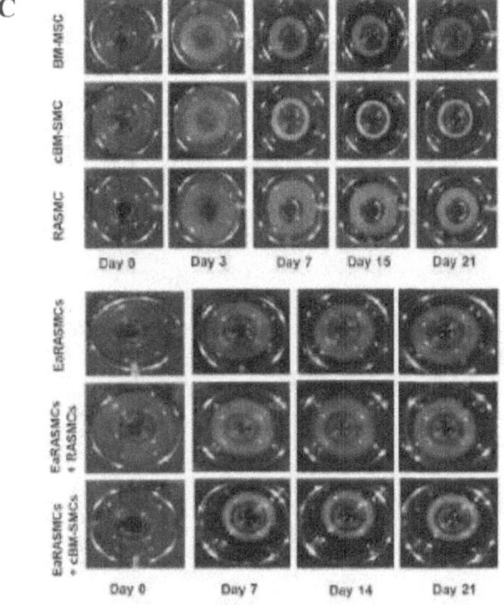

Figure 28. Gel Contraction over 21 days. (A) Quantitative analysis of contraction rate of collagen constructs seeded with standalone RASMCs, cBM-SMCs and BM-MSCs. * and # shows significance with respect to RASMCs and BM-MSCs respectively. (B) Quantitative analysis of contraction rate of collagen constructs seeded with standalone EaRASMCs, and co-culture of EaRASMCs with cBM-SMCs and RASMCs. * shows significance with respect to EaRASMCs deemed for p < 0.05. (C) and (D) Photographic image showing contraction of collagen gels in standalone and co-culture model respectively

4.3.2   Cell viability and proliferation

LIVE/DEAD staining of the constructs in all groups indicate the cells to be predominantly alive (stained green) with only sporadic dead cells (stained red), not limited to any one group (**Figure 29C**). Despite identically seeding the constructs in all groups, the DNA assay indicated significantly higher cell counts in the constructs seeded with the undifferentiated BM-MSCs relative to those seeded with the cBM-SMCs and healthy RASMCs; the RASMCs cultures appeared to proliferate the slowest (**Figure 29A**). Proliferation of the EaRASMCs over the same time period was

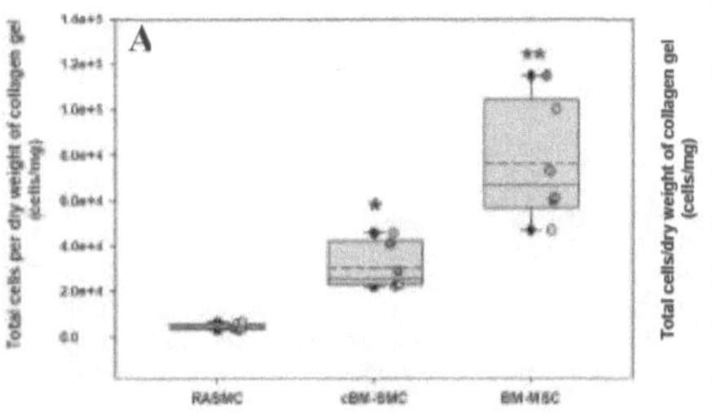

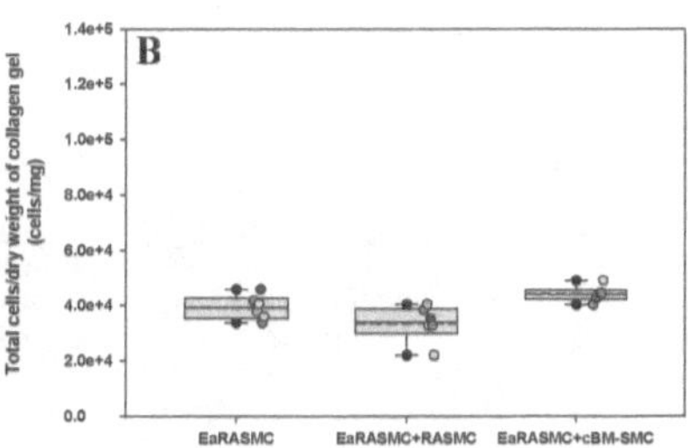

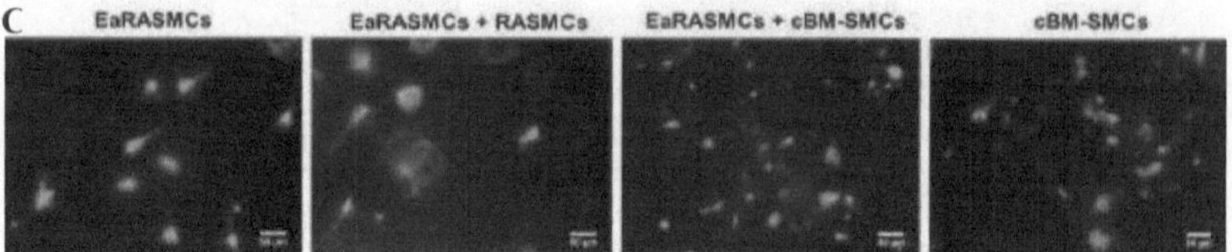

Figure 29. Cell proliferation and viability. (A) and (B) Cell proliferation within the collagen constructs as measured by DNA assay in standalone culture and co-culture respectively. Each color dots in the box plot represent the values for each replicate. Hence 6 colored dots show values for 6 replicates of each case and the blue dotted line shows the mean. * shows significance with respect to RASMCs and ** shows significance with respect to both RASMCs and cBM-SMCs respectively deemed for p < 0.05. (C) Cell viability within the collagen constructs as measured by live/dead assay. Scale Bar: 50um

intermediate between the RASMCs and cBM-SMCs. Co-culture with RASMCs or cBM-SMCs had no effect on total cell count within the constructs, as measured at 21 days of culture (**Figure 29B**).

4.3.3 Quantification of de novo elastic matrix synthesis within collagen constructs

The results of the FASTIN assay for measuring de novo synthesized elastic matrix, are shown in **Figures 30A and B.** In the constructs seeded with a single cell type, elastic matrix amounts per dry weight of constructs was significantly higher for the cBM-SMCs versus the RASMCs (p = 0.01). There were no significant differences in elastin synthesis between RASMCs and undifferentiated BM-MSCs (p = 0.05).

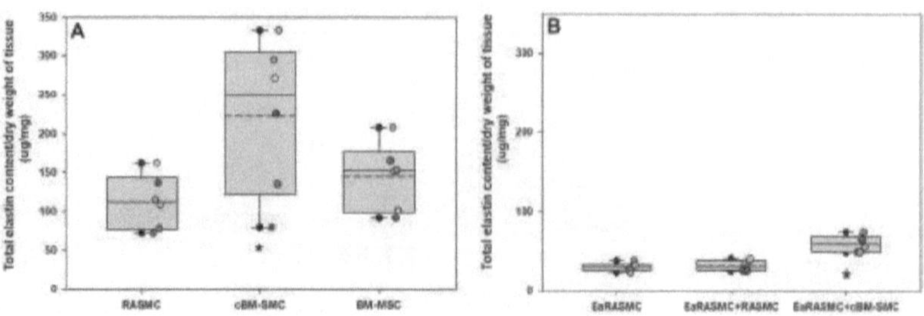

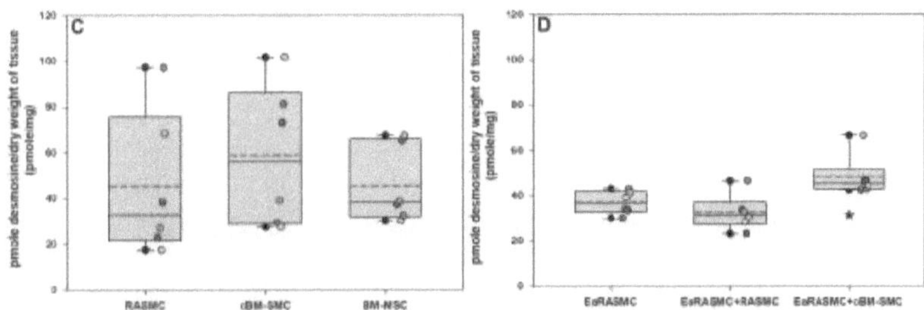

Figure 30. (A) and (B) Total elastin amount. Total elastin content (ug) produced by the cells per dry weight of construct as measured by FASTIN assay in standalone culture and co-culture respectively. (C) and (D) Total desmosine amount. Total desmosine content (pmole) produced by the cells per dry weight of construct as measured by ELISA assay in standalone culture and co-culture respectively. The box plot represents median (solid line) with 25/75% confidence interval; whiskers indicate 5/95% confidence interval; black circles indicate outliers and blue dashed lines indicate the mean. Each color dots in the box plot represent the values for each replicate. Hence 6 colored dots show values for 6 replicates of each case and the blue dotted lines shows the mean. * shows significance with respect to RASMCs or EaRASMCs

Elastic matrix synthesis by EaRASMCs was significantly lower than any of the other cell types **(Figure 30B)** but was significantly increased when co-cultured with cBM-SMCs (p= 0.000004) vs. EaRASMCs, but not upon co-culture with healthy RASMCs.

Figures 30C and D show desmosine crosslink content in the different culture groups, measured using ELISA. Desmosine content, normalized to construct dry weight was deemed not different between constructs seeded with RASMCs, cBM-SMCs and BM-MSCs **(Figure 30C).** Desmosine crosslinking of constructs seeded with EaRASMCs was significantly lower than in constructs containing RASMCs (p<0.001) cBM-SMCs (p<0.001) and BM-MSCs (p<0.001). Desmosine content, normalized to construct dry weight was significantly higher in co-cultures of the cBM-SMCs and EaRASMCs vs. constructs containing EaRASMCs alone (p = 0.02). On the other hand, desmosine content, normalized to construct dry weight in co-cultures of the cBM-SMCs and EaRASMCs was not different compared to constructs containing cocultured EaRASMCs and RASMCs **(Figure 30D)**.

4.3.4   Assessment of proteolysis within the collagen constructs

Western blots **(Figure 31A, 31B and 31C)** did not show significant differences in total, zymogen and active MMP-2 protein expression respectively within collagen constructs seeded with cBM-SMCs alone compared to constructs seeded with RASMCs alone and undifferentiated BM-MSCs alone. MMP-9 protein expression **(Figure 31D)** in cBM-SMC-seeded constructs and BM-MSC seeded constructs was significantly lower compared to constructs seeded with RASMCs alone (p ≤ 0.001) but was not different was seen compared to standalone BM-MSCs. Total, Zymogen and Active MMP-2 protein expression was not different measured in co-cultures of both EaRASMCs and RASMCs and EaRASMCs and cBM-SMCs versus constructs containing EaRASMCs alone **(Figure 31E, 31F and 31G)**. Similarly, MMP-9 protein expression was also not different in cocultures of both EaRASMCs and RASMCs and EaRASMCs and cBM-SMCs versus constructs containing EaRASMCs alone **(Figure 31H)**.

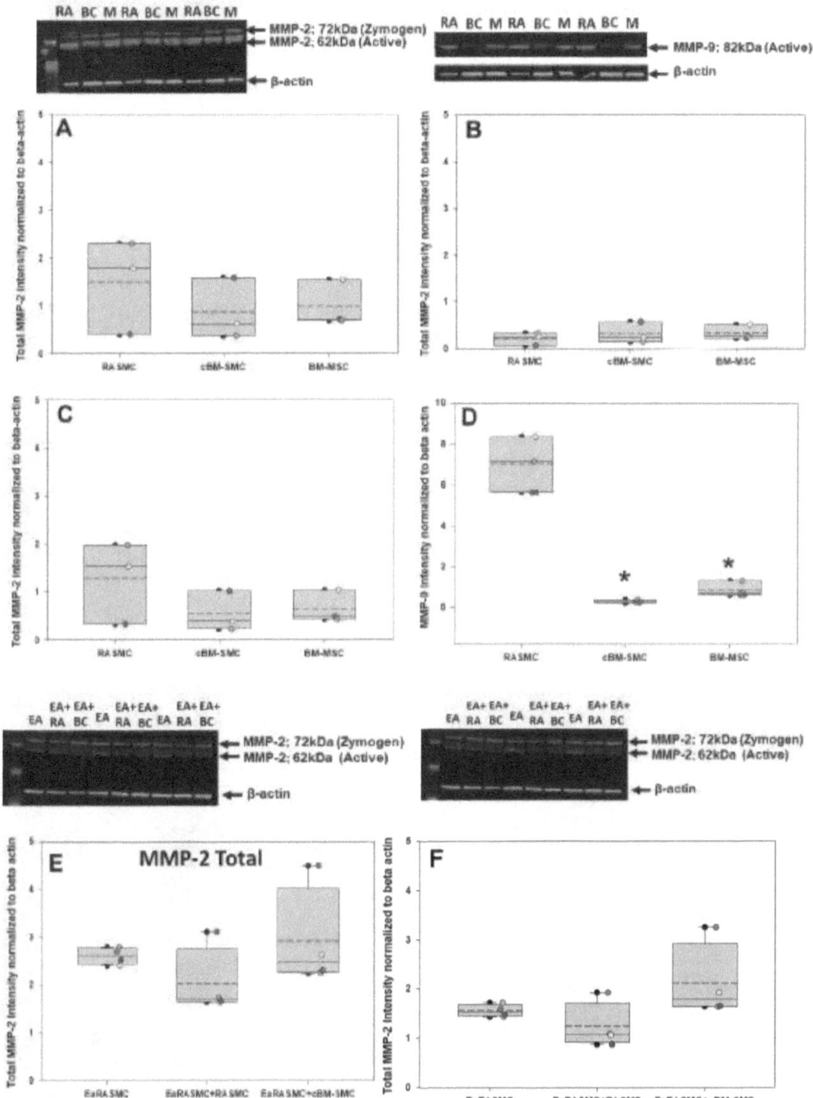
RA BC M RA BC M RA BC M
MMP-2; 72kDa (Zymogen)
MMP-2; 62kDa (Active)
β-actin
RA BC M RA BC M RA BC M
MMP-9; 82kDa (Active)
β-actin
A
Total MMP-2 intensity normalized to beta-actin
RA SMC
cBM-SMC
BM-MSC
B
Total MMP-2 intensity normalized to beta-actin
RA SMC
cBM-SMC
BM-MSC
C
Total MMP-2 intensity normalized to beta-actin
RA SMC
cBM-SMC
BM-MSC
D
MMP-9 intensity normalized to beta actin
RA SMC
cBM-SMC
BM-MSC
EA+ EA+ EA+ EA+ EA+ EA+
EA RA BC EA RA BC EA RA BC
MMP-2; 72kDa (Zymogen)
MMP-2; 62kDa (Active)
β-actin
EA+ EA+ EA+ EA+ EA+ EA+
EA RA BC EA RA BC EA RA BC
MMP-2; 72kDa (Zymogen)
MMP-2; 62kDa (Active)
β-actin
E
MMP-2 Total
Total MMP-2 intensity normalized to beta actin
EaRA SMC
EaRA SMC+RA SMC
EaRA SMC+cBM-SMC
F
Total MMP-2 intensity normalized to beta actin
EaRA SMC
EaRA SMC+RA SMC
EaRA SMC+cBM-SMC

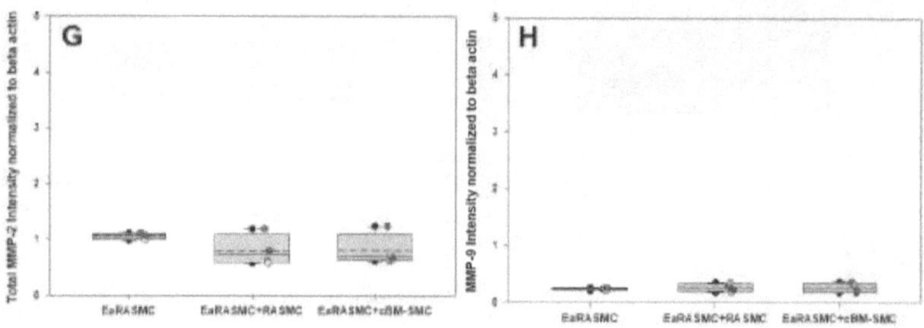

Figure 31: MMP-2 and MMP-9 protein expression. (A), (B), (C) and (D) Total, zymogen and active MMP-2 and active MMP-9 protein expression respectively in standalone culture. (E), (F), (G) and (H) Total, zymogen and active MMP-2 and active MMP-9 protein expression respectively in co-culture. * represents significance with respect to RASMC deemed for p < 0.05. The box plot represents median (solid line) with 25/75% confidence interval; whiskers indicate 5/95% confidence interval; black circles indicate outliers and blue dashed lines indicate the mean. Each color dots in the box plot represent the values for each replicate. Hence 3 colored dots show values for 3 replicates of each case and the blue dotted line shows the mean

4.3.5   Histological assessments of elastin content

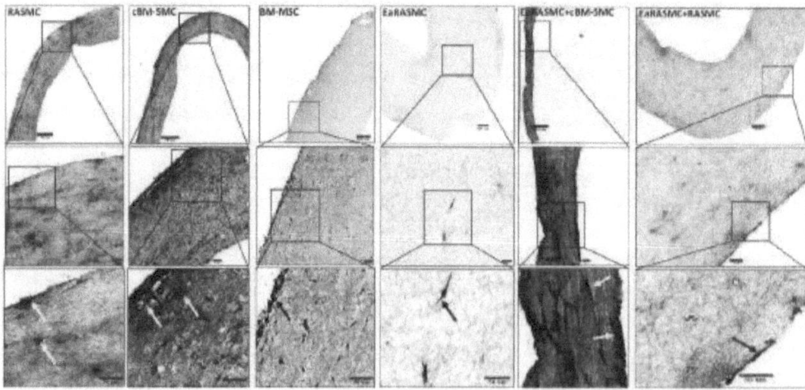

Figure 32: Histology of the cell seeded constructs. Paraffin embedded, VVG stained sections of cells seeded collagen gel constructs in different magnifications. Each column shows different types of cells seeded constructs. Black and white arrows in the third column point elastin fibers stained in dark blue or black. Scale bar: First row: 500 ums; second and third row: 50 um

Low and high magnification images of VVG-stained sections of the constructs in the different groups are shown in **Figure 32**.

Consistent with published literature [264], [265], in this uniaxial cell-compaction model of collagen, elastin deposition if noted, was significantly greater at the edges of the construct than in the bulk of the tissue. Morphometric analysis indicated no significant differences in elastin content (measured as percent area of elastin) between the standalone cultures of RASMCs, BM-MSCs and cBM-SMCs (**Figure 33A**). VVG staining indicated little or no detectable elastin in standalone EaRASMC cultures, which was the elastin among all groups tested (**Figure 33B**). While co-culture of RASMCs with EaRASMCs had no significant effect on elastic matrix deposition, the percent area of elastin was significantly higher in co-cultures of EaRASMCs and the cBM-SMCs (0.4 ± 0.3) (**Figure 33B**) vs. EaRASMCs alone (0 ± 0) (p = 0.003) and co-cultures of EaRASMCs and RASMCs (0.01 ± 0.001) (p = 0.007). Morphometry also indicated significantly lower minimal diameter of elastin deposits in standalone cultures of cBM-SMCs relative to cultures of RASMCs and BM-SMCs (p<0.001 and p=0.001) (**Figure 33C**). As expected, minimum diameter of elastin deposits in the co-cultures of EaRASMCs and both RASMCs and cBM-SMCs were much higher than in standalone EaRASMC cultures, (p < 0.001 in both the cases) (**Figure 33D**). The mean minimum diameter of elastin deposits in cocultures of EaARSMCs and RASMCs was modestly lower than in EaRASMC-cBM-SMC cocultures (2.8 ± 0.2 μm vs. 3 ± 0.2 μm; p = 0.02), though there were no differences between the co-culture groups.

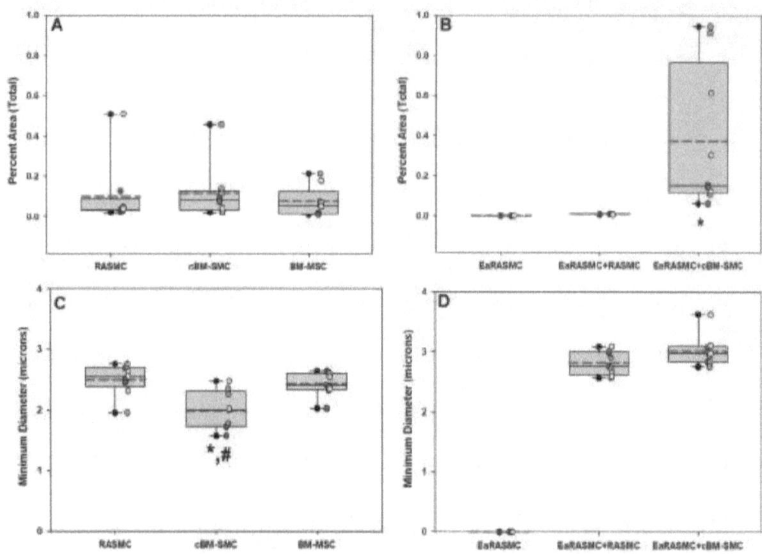

Figure 33: (A) and (B) Morphometry results. Total percent area (× 100%) of elastin in each construct as measured by morphometry in standalone culture and co-culture respectively. The box plot represents median (solid line) with 25/75% confidence interval; whiskers indicate 5/95% confidence interval; black circles indicate outliers and blue dashed lines indicate the mean. Each color dots in the box plot represent the values for each section. Data was collected from 3 constructs in each group with 3 histological sections per construct for a total of 9 sections. Each colored circle corresponds to sections from same construct. * represents significance with respect to EaRASMC deemed for p < 0.05. (C) and (D) Morphometry results. Minimum diameter of elastin fibers in each construct as measured by morphometry in standalone and co-culture respectively. The box plot represents median (solid line) with 25/75% confidence interval; whiskers indicate 5/95% confidence interval; black circles indicate outliers and blue dashed lines indicate the mean. Each color dots in the box plot represent the values for each section. Data was collected from 3 constructs in each group with 3 histological sections per construct for a total of 9 sections. Each colored circle corresponds to sections from same construct. * and # represent significance with respect to RASMCs and BM-MSC respectively deemed for p < 0.05

The visualization of VVG stained elastin was also confirmed by Pontamine sky blue labelling **(Figure 34)** which shows the similar pattern of elastin organization within the constructs as shown by VVG staining.

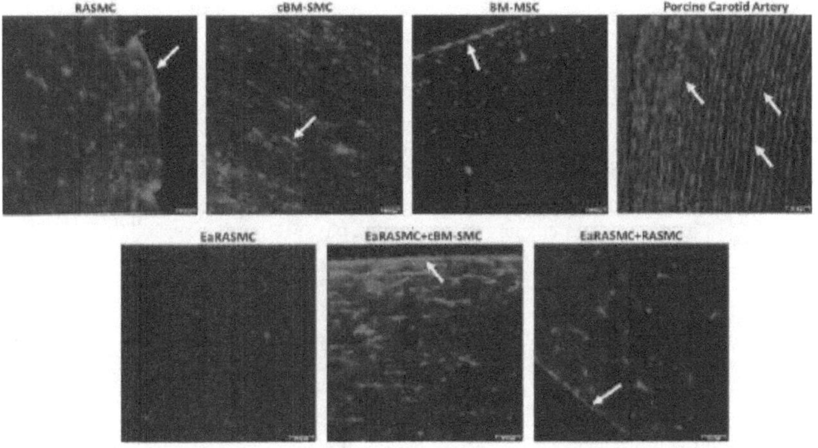

Figure 34: Autofluorescence of Elastin. Pontamine sky blue labelled constructs showing bright red auto fluorescence of elastin as indicated by white arrows. Scale bar: 70 um

4.4   Discussion

While our investigation of the AAA proposed treatment approach with non-human aneurysmal smooth muscle cells and stem cells is driven by the need to perform a first stage of preclinical testing in an animal model of AAAs, we have taken measures to support clinical relevance and future clinical translation of the generated findings.

In previous aim, we investigated how conditions of differentiation of rat BM-MSCs impacted phenotype of derived SMCs. We identified a set of conditions that generated SMCs of a non-terminally differentiated phenotype, that exhibit both a high level of contractility and yet high capacity for generating elastic matrix relative to even healthy rat aortic SMCs [257]. These derived SMCs, which we investigate further in this study as cBM-SMCs, were found to a) show distinct differences in protein expression profiles compared to EaRASMCs (see heat map of protein synthesis in (**Figure 35**), indicative their divergent phenotypes (see volcano plot in **Figure 35**), and b) provide paracrine pro-elastogenic and anti-proteolytic stimuli to rat aneurysmal SMCs (EaRASMCs) in non-contact 2-D co-cultures. Despite this promise, it is necessary to further investigate correlates of these pro-matrix regenerative effects of cBM-SMCs in a 3D microenvironment, in which cells are surrounded by other cells and matrix in 3 dimensions evocative of a physiologic milieu; such a 3-D culture milieu can thus more realistically simulate patterns of cell adherence, cytoskeletal organization, signal transduction, and contractile phenotypic state *in vivo*, and cellular response to treatments *in vivo*. While the ultimate validation of the efficacy of an approach to treat disease lies in testing the same *in vivo*, our current objective is to assess the elastic matrix regenerative and anti-proteolytic properties of cBM-SMCs which cannot be deduced from *in vivo* assessments which provide only gross changes to matrix homeostasis. Thus, in this aim, we investigated these aspects in an *in vitro* 3D cell-compacted collagen construct model, selected to simulate a de-elasticized, collagen rich AAA wall milieu.

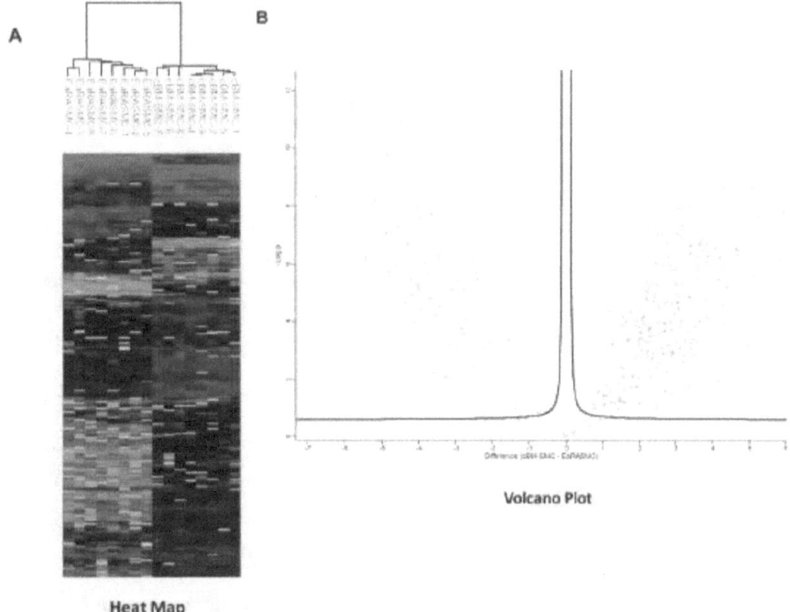

Figure 35: Proteomics analysis of cBM-SMCs and EaRASMCs. (A) Heat map showing difference in protein profile of cBM-SMCs and BM-MSCs. (B) Volcano plot showing the differential expression of proteins in EaRASMCs vs. cBM-SMCs

Results presented in **Figure 28** indicate significantly greater contractility of cBM-SMCs, versus healthy RASMCs, in a 3-D milieu. These results mirror trends we have observed in 2-D cultures as well [5]. This might be attributed to significantly higher expression of smooth muscle α-actin expression and myosin heavy chain II by cBM-SMCs versus RASMCs, which we previously reported [257]. It is known the upon contractile stimulation, proteins forming ECM adhesion complexes assemble at the cell membrane and trigger polymerization of actin filaments that in turn strengthen the membrane [266], a phenomenon that is more pronounced in actin-rich cells. This helps to transmit the forces due to the contractile mechanisms orchestrated by myosin heavy chain within the cell to the ECM, thus allowing the cells to adapt to mechanical stresses in their environment. While our prior studies did not indicate higher actin expression

106

[257] in undifferentiated BM-MSCs, and showed them to be less contractile than RASMCs in 2-D cultures, the significant contractility exhibited by BM-MSC-seeded constructs in **Figure 28** may be attributed to the rapid proliferation of these cells versus the other cell types (see **Figure 29A**), to result in much high cellularity and ECM compaction. Collagen constructs seeded with both EaRASMCs and cBM-SMCs also showed much greater contraction vs. constructs seeded with EaRASMCs alone and with EaRASMCs and RASMCs. Because a) cell seeding counts were identical in all cases, and b) total cellularity of constructs at 21 days were not different (**Figure 29B**) suggesting identical rates of overall cell proliferation, considering cell death was not an impacting factor (**Figure 29C**), the differences in contraction between the construct groups can be attributed solely to differences in contractility of component cell types. Also, the differences in the contraction profiles of constructs containing co-cultures of EaRASMCs and cBM-SMCs versus those containing cBM-SMCs alone suggest that tissue compaction is a function of the number of the primary contractile cells (cBM-SMCs).

Mirroring trends in our aim-1 2-D culture studies, in a 3-D collagenous milieu also, elastic matrix neo-assembly was significantly higher in cBM-SMC cultures versus RASMC cultures (**Figure 30A**). This can likely be attributed to significantly higher expression of elastic fiber assembly proteins such as fibulins 4 and 5, and of the elastin crosslinking enzyme, lysyl oxidase (LOX) we have measured in cBM-SMCs versus RASMCs [257]. As expected, elastic matrix synthesis in constructs seeded with EaRASMCs was significantly lower than even the RASMC-seeded constructs (**Figure 30B**). Co-culturing the EaRASMCs with cBM-SMCs but not RASMCs significantly increased elastic matrix deposition, a likely outcome of both the higher elastogenicity of the cBM-SMCs (**Figure 30A**) and possibly, based on our previous findings [6], stimulatory effects on elastogenesis by EaRASMCs.

Desmosine crosslink content within our constructs in cBM-SMC constructs was not different from that in the RASMC-seeded constructs in contradiction to our findings in 2-D culture [257]. In 2-D cultures of cBM-SMCs, de novo elastic matrix synthesis greatly exceeds that of collagen (>10: 1 w/w) and thus desmosine amounts normalized to total protein content of cultures are reliably indicative of desmosine crosslinking of the elastic matrix. Differently, within our 3-D constructs, the sum total of exogenous and newly synthesized collagen greatly exceeds the amount of cell-secreted matrix elastin. Hence, the desmosine amounts presented on a dry weight of tissue basis (**Figure 30C**) provides a comparison of total desmosine content and does not necessarily indicate extent of crosslinking of the elastic matrix alone. Further investigation using mass spectrometry analysis [267] is required to assess changes to crosslinking and elastin modifications in our samples. While overall desmosine synthesis in cBM- SMC seeded constructs was not different from that in EaRASMC-seeded constructs, desmosine amounts were modestly, but significantly higher in cocultures of EaRASMCs and cBM-SMCs, suggesting that the latter cells improve desmosine crosslinking of matrix elastin likely through their paracrine effects on their EaRASMCs.

Favorably, elastolytic MMPs specifically MMP-2 and MMP-9 (which specifically target elastic matrix degradation and are highly upregulated in AAAs, contributing to loss of vessel elasticity and AAA growth and whose inhibition has been linked to slowing or preventing AAA formation and slowing AAA growth) expression in cBM-SMC-seeded constructs was similar (MMP2) or lower (MMP9) than in the healthy RASMC-seeded constructs **(Figure 31)**, suggesting a less-activated SMC phenotype in 3D culture. MMP-2 expression in cBM-SMC containing co-cultures while apparently lower than in the other cases, was not deemed significantly different most likely due to the cells being pooled from multiple animals. In case of MMP-9, it is to be noted that we did not detect any MMP-9 zymogen although expression of active MMP-9 was significantly decreased in cBM-SMCs cultures vs RASMCs **(Figure 31G)**, suggesting lower MMP-9 activity. The lack of significant differences in expression of active MMP-9 between EaRASMC cultures and co-cultures of these cells with cBM-SMCs **(Figure 31H)** and separately, RASMCs may be attributed to lower expression in all cultures, at lower limit of detection. While the mechanisms underlying these outcomes need to be explored in future studies, we hypothesize that in general, higher compaction of constructs by cBM-SMCs leads to increased stiffness of the matrix, which in turn increases cytoskeletal tension to alter (reduce) MMP gene expression within these cells.

Histological assessments of elastic matrix through VVG-staining **(Figure 32)** was highly consistent with findings from the Fastin analysis. The results showed significantly greater compaction of constructs and resultant higher cellular density and increased elastic matrix deposition by cBM-SMCs relative to BM-MSCs and RASMCs. The cBM-SMCs also clearly increased these outcomes in constructs containing EaRASMCs, which by alone produced very little elastic matrix. As seen in both the VVG-stained sections and in pontamine sky-blue treated sections, except in constructs containing cBM-SMCs, elastin deposition in other cases was mostly limited to the edges of the construct, a phenomenon we have reported in earlier work [231]. This may be attributed to high stress gradients that exist along the construct edges, which stimulates elastogenesis by cells. Elastic matrix in the interior of the constructs, where observed, was mostly in the form of amorphous elastin clumps. Differently, in constructs containing cBM-SMCs alone or in co-culture with EaRASMCs, significant elastic fiber assembly was noted in the interior and edges of cBM-SMC and cBM-SMC/EaRASMC constructs. This may be attributed to higher expression of key elastic fiber assembly proteins such as fibulins by cBM-SMCs, which we have previously shown [257], and in standalone cBM-SMC cultures, also to lower activity of elastolytic MMP2. Quantitative assessment of VVG stained sections using morphometry **(Figure 33)** confirmed the results of FASTIN assay in showing significantly higher percent area of elastin in constructs containing both EaRASMCs and cBM-SMCs relative to EaRASMCs alone, and EaRASMCs and RASMCs together. The results indicate that EaRASMCs do not produce much elastin on their own, but are stimulated by cBM-SMCs, likely via their paracrine secretions, to greatly increase elastic matrix deposition. Again, such effects were not seen with co-culture of the EaRASMCs with RASMCs. Co-culture cBM-SMC but not RASMC is inciting elastin formation by the EaRASMCs. The diameter of mature elastic fibers are in the range of 0.5 to 1.5 microns [268]. A significantly higher diameter of the elastin deposits was noted in constructs containing RASMCs (2.5 ± 0.2 microns) and separately, BM-MSC (2.4 ± 0.2 microns) versus constructs containing cBM-SMC (1.9 ± 0.3 microns). In cBM-SMC cultures, it is certainly possible that elastin fibrils are closely appositioned by significant contraction of the construct to form a mature fiber, whereas in the RASMC and BM-MSC cultures, poor contraction of the constructs results in a more diffuse cluster of elastin fibrils exhibiting higher cluster diameters. While co-culture of EaRASMCs with CBM-SMCs and separately RASMCs, greatly increased elastic matrix accumulation within the constructs, the diameters of the elastin deposits in the latter cultures was higher (3 ± 0.2

microns and 2.8 ± 0.2 microns) than that which might be expected for a mature elastic fiber. This might be attributed to high expression of MMPs by EaRASMCs, a milieu in which re-clustering of elastin occurs into aggregates. The re-clustering of elastin into these aggregates may be incited by abnormal accumulation of glycoprotein (fibrillin) microfibrils (pre-scaffolds onto which crosslinked elastin aggregates coalesce to form fibers) during elastolysis in the presence of MMPs, as has been reported in literature [269].

In summary, the outcomes of this aim demonstrate significant potential benefits of cBM-SMCs to augmenting elastic matrix neo-assembly and fiber formation, and attenuating proteolysis in a 3D, collagenous milieu evocative of the de-elasticized aneurysm wall, which proffers attractive prospects for use in cell therapies for AAA wall repair. We acknowledge that further studies are required to further determine the relative contributions of new elastic matrix assembly by cBM-SMCs and their pro-elastogenic effects on EaRASMCs to the observed increases in elastic fiber assembly in cBM-SMC/EaRASMC co-cultures. Rigorous proteomic assessments of cBM-SMCs and EaRASMCs are also required to ascertain key differences in protein expression that account for, or alternately, might result from differences in their phenotype, and to identify secreted factors necessary and sufficient for the pro-elastogenic and anti-proteolytic effects of the cBM-SMCs. Also, potentially critical to the effectiveness of the treatment approach *in vivo* is the need to localize the cBM-SMCs at the AAA tissue site and accordingly necessity to assess their ability to home into the injured tissue as BM-MSCs have been shown to do [270], following systemic delivery. Alternately, the ability of our derived SMCs to provide therapeutic benefit through long-range paracrine signaling from remote site would also assure their therapeutic utility. These aspects critical to clinical translation of our cell therapy approach will be described in next

chapter.

CHAPTER V

ASSESSING FATE, SAFETY, AND AAA REPERATIVE EFFECTS OF BM-MSC AND cBM-SMC *IN VIVO*

5.1 Introduction

Cell therapy represents interventions wherein viable cells of one or more types are either infused/injected, implanted, or engrafted into a recipient in order to elicit a therapeutic effect. This approach has shown promise in recent years in restoring the lost function of damaged tissues or organs [271]. Diverse autologous, allogeneic, and xenogeneic cell types including resident stem cells (SCs) and stem cell precursors, multipotent adult progenitor cells, embryonic stem cells, pancreatic islet cells, and others have been leveraged for cell therapy [272]. Such therapies have been applied to stabilize or even reverse conditions such as diabetes, neurodegenerative diseases (Parkinsons, Alzheimers), cardiovascular diseases (myocardial infarction, atherosclerosis, aortic aneurysms) and for islet transplantation for pancreas [272].

Recent evidence strongly suggests involvement of SCs and SC-derived smooth muscle cells (SMCs) in vascular morphogenesis [273], [274] and tissue repair after injury [275] which are the only physiologic scenarios in the vasculature wherein elastic matrix is prolifically synthesized. These outcomes, and the promise of these cells for stimulating tissue repair have prompted us to hypothesize that they will be effective in restoring matrix homeostasis in the AAA wall to slow, arrest or even reverse AAA pathophysiology. Recent preclinical and clinical studies have shown high promise of mesenchymal stem cells (MSCs), which are multipotent adult stem cells, for tissue repair and functional restoration *in vivo*. As discussed in Chapter II, MSCs are likely suited to such applications due to (a) well documented phenotype and characteristics for effective quality control, (b) easy accessibility [276], (c) simple and well-defined processes for isolation and scale up for clinical use [277], (d) ease of preservation with minimal loss of viability and potency, and (e) no adverse effects upon allogenic transplantation making it easier to find donors in case of critical patients [278]. Bone marrow MSCs (BM-MSCs) have also been shown to have the capacity for multi-lineage differentiation, including into SMCs, as we have shown in a prior chapters, which can be leveraged to develop cell-based approaches for *in vivo* cardiovascular regeneration and *in vitro* tissue engineering. Finally, MSCs have been demonstrated to possess anti-inflammatory and immune suppressive properties and the capacity to naturally home into the diseased site to impart the desired reparative benefits [5]. In a previous body of work from our lab, we investigated the pro-elastogenic effects of MSCs and their derivatives and their ability to augment elastin matrix synthesis by resident aneurysmal SMCs towards reversing proteolytic damage to the ECM, particularly the elastic matrix, which is a major cause of continual aortal expansion in AAAs. We demonstrated success in differentiating MSCs into SMC like cells of specific phenotypes exhibiting both high elastogenicity, anti-proteolytic properties, and high contractility *in vitro* [5], [6]. Collectively, these findings motivate us to investigate the *in vivo* tissue reparative effects of BM-MSCs and their SMC derivatives (cBM-SMCs) in the context of AAA treatment in a rat model of the disease.

While we have shown in chapter III that our differentiated cBM-SMCs retain their phenotype and superior elastogenicity in long term culture, major issues associated with cell therapy such as their ability to home in to the AAA tissue following minimally invasive method intravenous delivery, their *in-vivo* bio distribution and retention in the AAA wall, and possible paracrine effects on AAA tissue repair processes even in the event of localization in remote tissues remain uncertain. In this chapter we describe studies that sought to investigate the natural homing of cBM-SMCs and their bio-distribution upon intravenous injection of bolus of cells on elastase infused rat AAA model. We also sought to establish the initial evidence of therapeutic potential of these cells in restoring elastin homeostasis and arresting AAA growth *in-vivo*.

5.2   Materials and Methods

5.2.1   mRNA isolation and RT PCR for homing receptor gene expression

The BM-MSCs were seeded in polystyrene 6-well plate (USA Scientific, Ocala, FL, USA) and cBM-SMCs were seeded in human Fn-coated 6-well plate (BD Biosciences, San Jose, CA, USA) at 15,000 cells per well ($A = 10$ cm^2). To study the effect of TNF-α stimulation on homing receptor gene expression, on day 14 of culture, the cells were serum starved for 3 hours with DMEM/F-12 containing 2% v/v FBS and 1% v/v PS. Following serum starvation, the cells were incubated with 0.1, 1 and 10 ng/ml of TNF- α for 24 hours and harvested in RLT buffer containing 1% v/v β-mercaptoethanol. As described in chapter II, total RNA was isolated from the cultures using a RNeasy mini kit (Qiagen, Valencia, CA, USA) and quantified using a Quant-iT™ Ribogreen® RNA kit (Invitrogen) following the manufacturer's instructions. An iScript cDNA synthesis kit (Bio-Rad, Hercules, CA, USA) was used to synthesize cDNA using 1 µg of RNA from all the samples and reverse transcription was performed for total of 40 minutes combining 5 minutes at 25 ˚C, 30 minutes at 42 ˚C and 5 minutes at 85 ˚C according to the manufacturer's instructions. Real time PCR was performed using an Applied Biosystems 7500 Real-Time PCR system with Power SYBR® Green Master Mix (Applied Biosystems). Specially designed primer was used for the 18s, the house - keeping gene (relatimeprimers.com) [Forward 5' to 3': CGGACAGGATTGACAGATTG and Reverse 5' to 3': ACGCCACTTGTCCCTC TAAG] and readymade primers was used for CXCR4 (Bio-Rad, Hercules, CA, USA; unique assay id# qRnoCED0007227) and CCR3 (Bio-Rad, Herculed, CA, USA; unique assay id# qRnoCED0055609). The PCR data was analyzed using LinReg PCR program as described in chapter II. This program uses a MATLAB® code separately for each sample to determine baseline-corrected set of values and window of linearity. PCR efficiency was calculated from the slope of linear fit for each sample. This provided correction for N0. Data value obtained from this analysis was directly used to calculate gene expression ratio as described in literature. A two-way ANOVA with Tukey multiple comparison was used for statistical significance.

5.2.2 Western Blot for homing receptor expression

Western blot analysis was performed to semi-quantitatively compare protein expression for the homing receptors CXCR4 and CCR3 for BM-MSC and cBM-SMCs. Briefly, the cells were seeded at a density of 30,000/well in a 6 well plate (n = 6 wells/case) and cultured for 21 days. To study the effect of TNF-α on homing receptor expression, as described above in section 1, at day 21 of culture, the cells were incubated with 0.1, 1 and 10 ng/ml of TNF-α for 24 hours following 3 hours of serum starvation. The cell layers were harvested in RIPA buffer containing a protease inhibitor cocktail (Thermo Scientific, Waltham, MA). The amount of protein in each sample was quantified using Pierce™ BCA assay kit (Thermo Scientific, Waltham, MA, USA). Western blotting was performed as described in chapter 3. Briefly, 15 ug of protein sample for both cell types were mixed with loading buffer. The mixture was reduced and loaded along with a pre-stained molecular weight ladder (Invitrogen) on to 4-12% SDS-PAGE. The gels were subjected to dry transfer onto nitrocellulose membranes using iBlot® western blotting system (Invitrogen). The membranes were then blocked with Odyssey blocking buffer (LiCOR Biosciences, Lincoln, NE, USA) for 1 hour at room temperature, and then incubated overnight with anti-CXCR4 antibody (Abcam, Cambridge, UK; # ab124824) and anti-CCR3 antibody (Abcam, Cambridge, UK; # ab32512) in manufacturer's recommended dilution. Following this, the blots were incubated with secondary antibodies against rabbit and mouse conjugated with IRDye® 680LT (1:15000 dilution) and IRDye® 800 CW (1:20000 dilution) respectively. The bands were observed using a LiCOR Odyssey laser-based scanning system, quantified using Image Studio™ Lite software as relative density units (RDU) normalized to the intensity the housekeeping protein (β-actin) bands. A two-way ANOVA with Tukey multiple comparison was used for statistical significance.

5.2.3   Immunofluorescence (IF) to visualize expression of homing receptor proteins

MSC homing receptors CXCR4 and CCR3 were detected by IF labeling, as described previously [228]. Cells were seeded on 12 well plates, cultured for 7 days, serum starved for 3 hours and incubated with different doses of TNF-α for 24 hours as described in **sections 5.2.1 and 5.2.2 above**. The cells were then were fixed using 4% w/v paraformaldehyde for 20 min at 4 °C and blocked with PBS containing 5% v/v goat serum (Gibco Life Technologies, Grand Island, NY, USA) for 20 minutes at room temperature. The cells were then incubated overnight with primary antibodies against the CXCR4 (Abcam, Cambridge, UK; # ab197203) and CCR3 (Abcam, Cambridge, UK; # ab32512). The expression of these proteins was then visualized using secondary antibodies conjugated to AlexaFluor 488 or 633 probes (Molecular Probes, Temecula, CA, USA). The cells were then incubated with aqueous DAPI (4', 6-Diamidine-2'-phenylindole dihydrochloride), the nuclear dye (Sigma Aldrich, St. Louis, MO, USA) at 1:10000 dilution for 30 mins at room temperature followed by multiple washing. Imaging was done using Leica SP8 confocal microscope (Leica Microsystems, Wetzlar, Germany) and the images were analyzed using the NIH- Image J® software. A two-way ANOVA with Tukey multiple comparison was used for statistical significance.

5.2.4   Generating small AAAs in rat model

All animal procedures were conducted with approval of the Institutional Animal Care and Use Committee (IACUC) at the Cleveland Clinic (ARC # 2019-2107). The animal facility at Cleveland Clinic is AAALAC-approved (animal assurance # A3145-01). AAAs were induced in male Sprague Dawley rats (Young Adult, 100-2120 g,

Charles River Laboratory, Wilmington, MA, USA) according to the established protocol of the Ramamurthi Lab using intraluminal elastase infusion method. Briefly, the rats were anesthetized using 2% v/v isoflurane (Piramal Enterprises Limited, Telangana, India). The rat was then placed in supine position on the surgical bench with continuous flow of anesthesia and the abdominal area was shaved and sterilized with Iodine and 70% alcohol pad. Following subcutaneous Bupivicaine injection (local anesthetic), the infrarenal aorta was then surgically exposed by laparotomy and clamped just below and just above the renal and iliac bifurcation respectively to occlude the blood flow. The clamped segment of the aorta was slowly infused with 40U/ml porcine pancreatic elastase (MP Biomedicals, Solon, USA; # 100617) and allowed to sit for 30 mins. After 30 mins the clamps were removed, blood flow was restored, and the intestines were replaced. The incision at muscle and dermal layer were closed with 4-0 Vicryl suture (Ethicon, Somerville, NJ) and 4-0 Monosof suture (Covidien, Dublin, Ireland) respectively. As the post-operative care, Buprenorphine injection was administered twice daily for 48 hours for pain management. The aneurysm was allowed to develop over the period of 3 weeks. AAA induction parameters were optimized so that the diameter did not exceed a 50% increase over the baseline diameter. This criterion ensured that our aneurysmal expansions are consistent with the % aortal size increases typical of the small AAAs in clinical patients, that we propose to treat by cell therapy in the future. The aneurysmal SMCs (EaRASMCs) used in chapter 4 were isolated from the aorta of these rats using an explant culture method as previously described.

5.2.5 Characterization of AAAs using small animal Magnetic Resonance Imaging (MRI)

AAA development as well as the effect of cell injection on the aorta in terms of size was characterized non-invasively using a small animal MRI (7T, Bruker Biospin Corp., Billerica, USA) using established method of our lab. Scanning was performed just prior to surgery to measure the baseline aortal volume and subsequent scannings were performed at 3 weeks post-surgery, 1 week after cell injection and 2 weeks after cell injection. For MRI, the rats were anesthetized in 2% v/v isoflurane as described above and positioned in pronation position in a BioSpec 70/20 Bruker USR MRI system with abdominal region aligned at the center of the magnetic field of the MR coil. Phase contrast angiography (PCA) scans were used to visualize the aorta. PCA basically scans the moving fluid or blood without requiring the contrast agents so as to obtain the images of major blood vessels of the body including the aorta. PCA relies on the principle that spins that are moving along the direction of magnetic field gradient develop a phase shift which is proportional to the velocity of the spins. Two gradients of equal magnitude and opposite direction are used to encode the velocity of the spins. Stationary spins arising from the stationary tissues do not undergo net change in the phase after applying the two equal and opposite gradients but the moving spins arising from the moving blood flow will experience a net phase shift. This phase shift information can be used directly to produce an angiogram.

Volumetric analysis of the scans was performed after imaging to obtain the volume changes in the abdominal aorta subjected to AAA induction or cell treatment post AAA formation. A 3-D rendering of the aorta was done using the software Microview Parallax™ (Parallax Innovations, Ontario, Canada) by subtracting the background to isolate the aorta and vena cava. The aneurysmal segment of the aorta and the number of slices within the segment were identified for the sequential scans of each animal to analyze the equal segment length for each animal. The volume was measured by tracing the contours of the circumference of the aortal segment in transverse plane along the length of the aorta at every 5 slices. The percentage change in volume between the baseline and AAA and baseline and treated aorta was plotted. Two-way RM-ANOVA was used to compare the statistical significance between the groups with Tukey multiple comparison where applicable for each doses and two-way ANOVA with Tukey multiple comparison was used to compare the effect of dose and effect of time between the groups and within the groups.

5.2.6 Labeling and intravenous injection of cells

BM-MSCs and cBM-SMCs were propagated in culture as described earlier. To visualize the biodistribution of cells *in vivo*, the cells were labeled with Vivo track 680 (Perkin Elmer, Waltham, USA; for 24 hours bio-distribution studies) and LuminiCell Tracker™ 670 Cell Labelling Kit (EMD Millipore, Burlington, MA; for 2 weeks biodistribution studies) following the manufacturers' protocol. Briefly, for labeling cells with Vivo track 680, the cells were trypsinized with 0.05% v/v trypsin (Media core, Cleveland Clinic) and 2.1×10^6 cells were resuspended in 400 ul of PBS. The aliquot of reconstituted Vivo track 680 was added to 400 ul of cell suspension and incubated for 20 mins at 37 °C in a shaker. Following incubation, the cells were washed 3 times for 10 mins each with DMEM/F-12 containing 10% v/v FBS. After the final wash the cells were resuspended in 750 ul of warm PBS and injected into the rats via tail vein injection. Similarly, for labelling cells with LuminiCell Tracker™ 680, the cells were trypsinized as mentioned above and 2.1×10^6 were resuspended in 1 ml of 2 nM LuminiCell Tracker™ 680 prepared in serum free DMEM/F-12 and incubated for 1 hour at 37 °C on a shaker. Following incubation, the cells were washed (2 cycles of 10 mins each) with DMEM/F-12 containing10% v/v FBS. The cells were then resuspended in 750 ul of warm PBS and injected into the rat via the tail vein. The schematic below shows the time of the experimental interventions:

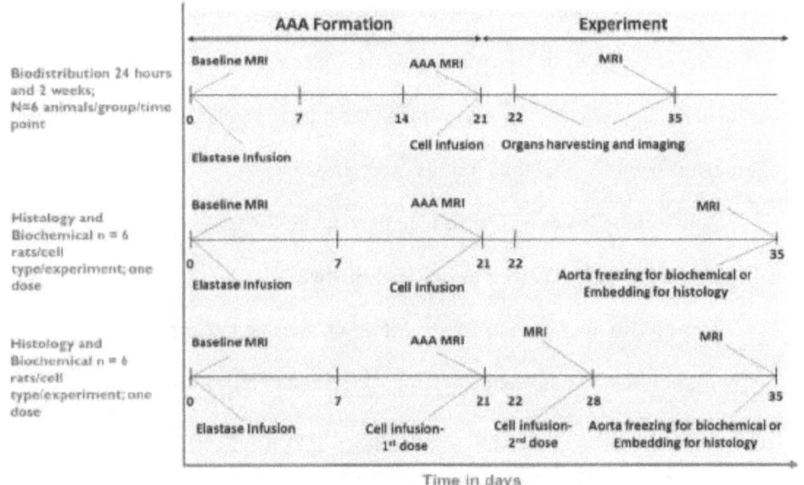

Figure 36: Experimental timeline

To visualize the distribution of cells *in vivo*, both at 24 hours and 2 weeks, the respective rats were euthanized using CO_2 asphyxiation and major organs (Lungs, Heart, Aorta, Liver, Kidneys and Spleen) were harvested. The organs were imaged with an IVIS Spectrum CT (Perkin Elmer, Waltham, USA) with machine-defined settings for the Vivo Track 680 ($\lambda = 675$ nm excitation, $\lambda = 720$ nm emission) and recommended settings for the LuminiCell Tracker 680 ($\lambda = 500$ to 535 nm excitation, $\lambda = 660$ to 680 nm emission). The sequence of images was then analyzed using Living Image Software™ (Perkin Elmer, Waltham, USA). Basically, each of the organs of the labeled cell-injected rats and PBS-injected control rats were imaged together and total radiant efficiency of each set of organs were measured. Total radiant efficiency is defined as sum of fluorescence emission radiance per excitation power ($[p/s]/[\mu W/cm^2]$). The average of total radiant efficiency of each organs of PBS injected rats were subtracted from the total radiant efficiency value of the each of the corresponding organs of the labeled cell-injected rats to obtain the background subtracted total radiant efficiency corresponding to the fluorescence signal from the probe. The background subtracted average signals for 6 separate organs were plotted. For organs like kidneys, where the total radiant efficiency was lower than the total radiant efficiency of background (PBS treated control), the final values were negative. A two-way ANOVA with Tukey multiple comparison was performed to compare the statistical significance between 24 hours and 2 weeks as well as between the two cell types for each organ whereas one-way ANOVA was used to compare the statistical significance between all the organs sepaartely for 24 hours and 2 weeks using Sigma Plot 13.0 software.

5.2.7   ELISA to assess C3 complement activation in plasma

C3 complement generation in plasma following the injection of cells was measured using a C3 complement ELISA kit (Abcam, Cambridge, UK, # ab157737) according to the manufacturer's protocol. C3 complement activation was measured after 24 hours and 2 weeks of cells injection. Plasma was isolated following the protocol adapted from Lee et.al[277]. Briefly, the rat was anesthetized as described above and laid down in a prone position on the surgical table with continuous flow of anesthesia. The rat's tail was slightly immersed in warm water to dilate the blood vessel as well as to make it visible. Blood was drawn from the lateral tail vein using a heparin coated

25G needle and collected in EDTA coated phlebotomy tube and was centrifuged at 2100×g and 4 °C for 15 mins. A clear layer of plasma separated out and RBC was settled on the bottom of the tube. The plasma was collected in a 1.5ml centrifuge tube and stored at -80 °C to maintain the complement activity.

For ELISA, the plasma was diluted 1:10000 v/v and the standards were prepared by serial dilution according to manufacturer's instructions (Abcam, Cambridge, UK, # ab157737). Both samples and standards were added to each well of the antibody coated strips and incubated for 20 mins at room temperature. Following incubation, the strips were washed 4 times and a 1× solution og Enzyme-Antibody Conjugate was added to each well and incubated for 20 mins in the dark at room temperature. The wash steps were repeated, and the reaction was stopped using stop solution. The absorbance of each well was measured at $\lambda = 450$ nm. A four-parameter algorithm (4PL) was used to plot the standard curve in order to determine the best fit. The C3 protein concentration was extrapolated using the standard curve. One-way ANOVA was used to compare the statistical significance between the groups both at 24 hours as well as 2 weeks.

5.2.8 Cytokine array

The change in proteome profile following cell injections was broadly assessed by a Proteome Profiler™ Array (R&D systems, Minneapolis, USA; # ARY030) per the manufacturer's instructions. Aortae from all the rats were harvested as described above after 2 weeks of cell injection. For healthy controls, aorta was obtained from healthy, age-matched rats. The aortal tissue was manually grinded in liquid nitrogen and incubated in RIPA buffer for 20 mins on ice. The samples were then homogenized by sonicating on ice. The samples were then centrifuged at full speed for 15 mins in 4 °C. The supernatant was collected and the protein samples from 6 rats were pooled for each of the cases. The concentration of pooled protein samples was determined using Pierce™ BCA protein assay kit. To perform the cytokine analysis, the cytokine array membrane was blocked for 1 hour at room temperature on a rocking platform using the provided blocking buffer. Each membrane was then incubated overnight at 4 °C with 200 µg of respective pooled protein samples for each of the cases. After overnight incubation, the blots were washed (3 cycles, 10 mins each) incubated with a primary antibody cocktail for 1 hour at room temperature. The wash step was repeated, and the blots were incubated with 1× Streptavidin-HRP for 30 mins at room temperature. The blots were washed again as previously described and 1ml of chemiluminescent reagent was added and allowed to rest for 1min. The blots were then exposed in a GE Amersham 600 Gel Imager (GE healthcare, Chicago, Illinois) in an auto exposure mode. The pixel density of each of the cytokines in duplicate were measured with NIH Image J™ software. The average of duplicate values was plotted for each cytokine.

5.2.9   Western blot analysis of aortal wall tissues

Western blots were used to measure expression of key proteins involved in elastin homeostasis in the aorta wall after 2 weeks of cell injection. Aorta tissue sample was collected and processed as described in **section 5.2.8** above. The protein content in the aortal tissue isolate from each rat was measured using a Pierce™ BCA protein assay kit and western blots was performed as described in **section 5.2.2** above. The list of antibodies used for each of the proteins are given in **Table V** below. Two-way ANOVA was used to compare the statistical significance between the groups.

Table V: List of antibodies

Protein	Host	Catalog #	Company
MMP-2	Rabbit	ab97779	Abcam
MMP-9	Rabbit	ab38898	Abcam
TIMP-1	Rabbit	ab61224	Abcam
LOX	Rabbit	ab31238	Abcam
JNK	Rabbit	ab208035	Abcam
Fibulin-5	Rabbit	ab202977	Abcam
TIMP-2	Rabbit	ab180630	Abcam
Fibulin-4	Rabbit	PA-544321	Thermo Scientific
SDF-1	Rabbit	NBP2-29480	Novus Biologicals
ERK-1/2	Rabbit	9102	Cell Signalling

5.3 Results

5.3.1 Gene expression for homing receptors

Gene expression for CXCR4 was significantly higher for cBM-SMCs vs BM-MSCs at unprimed and 0.1 ng/ml of TNF-α. While no difference was seen in CXCR4 gene expression by BM-MSCs with TNF-α priming, cBM-SMCs had significantly higher CXCR4 gene expression for unprimed vs 10 ng/ml, 0.1 ng/ml vs 10 ng/ml and significantly lower for unprimed vs 0.1 ng/ml **(Figure 37A)**. CCR3 expression was significantly higher in cBM-SMCs vs BM-MSCs for 0.1 ng/ml and 1ng/ml of TNF-α. Like CXCR4, no difference was seen in CCR3 expression by BM-MSC with priming, cBM-SMCs showed significantly higher CCR3 expression for 0.1 ng/ml vs unprimed, 1 ng/ml and 10 ng/ml **(Figure 37B)**.

5.3.2 Expression of homing receptor proteins

No difference was seen in CXCR4 protein expression between cBM-SMCs and BM-MSCs as well as no effect of priming was seen for both the cell types **(Figure 38A)**. In contrary, CCR3 protein expression was significantly higher in cBM-SMCs in all doses of TNF-α whereas no effect of priming was seen within the cell types **(Figure 38B)**.

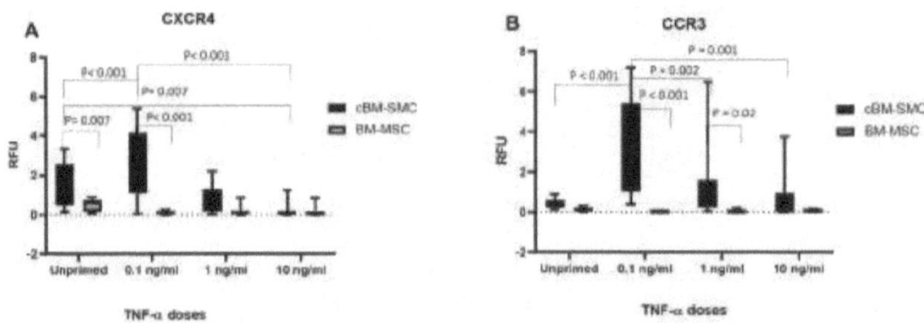

Figure 37. (A) and (B) CXCR4 and CCR3 gene expression by BM-MSC and cBM-SMC respectively

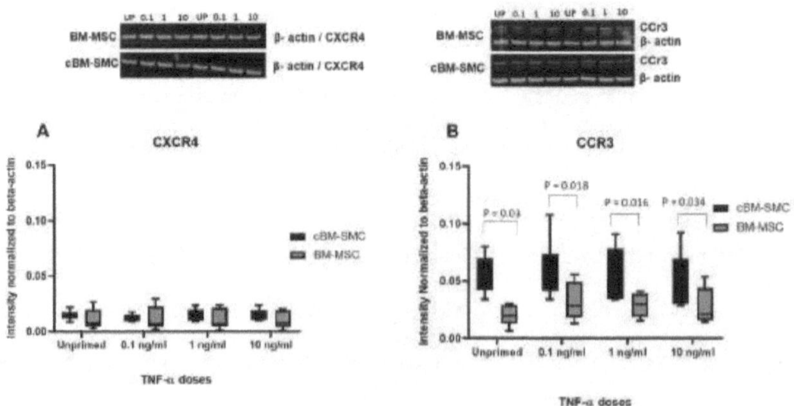

Figure 38. (A) and (B) CXCR4 and CCR3 protein expression by BM-MSC and cBM-SMC respectively

5.3.3 Immunofluorescence expression of homing receptors

Immunofluorescence staining showed significantly higher expression of both CXCR4 and CCR3 proteins by cBM-SMCs vs BM-MSCs **(Figure 39 C and D)**. While no difference was seen in CXCR4 expression by BM-MSCs with priming cBM-SMCs showed significantly higher CXCR4 expression for 0.1 ng/ml vs unprimed, 1 ng/ml and 10 ng/ml of TNF-α. Similarly, for CCR3 no effect of priming was seen in BM-MSCs, however, cBM-SMCs showed significantly higher expression at 1 ng/ml vs unprimed, 0.1ng/ml and 10 ng/ml of TNF-α.

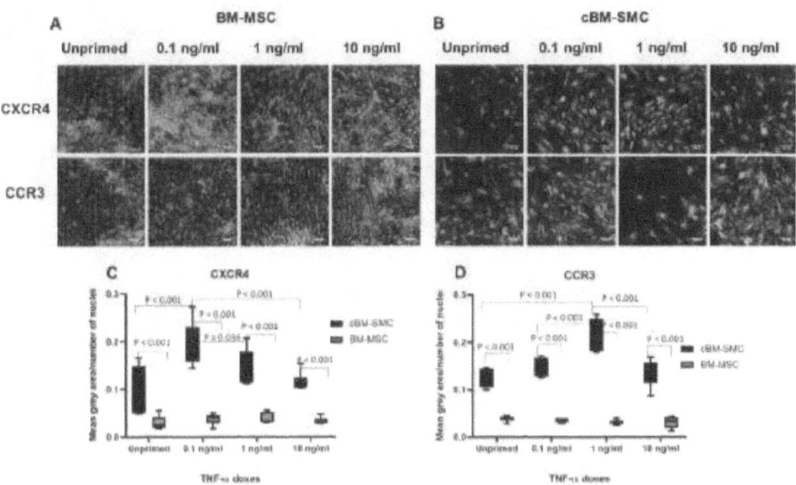

Figure 39. (A) and (B) Immunofluorescence staining showing CXCR4 and CCR3 expression by BM-MSCs and cBM-SMCs. Blue: nuclei and Green: homing receptors (CXCR4/CCR3) (C) and (D) Quantification of target protein radiant density normalized to number of nuclei

5.3.4   Short and long-term biodistribution of cells *in vivo*

Figure 40 shows the cell-associated fluorescence as well as the auto fluorescence seen in each of the 6 organs for each of the cell treated cases and PBS treated controls. The biodistribution of cells as estimated from the total radiant efficiency also defined as sum of fluorescence emission radiance per excitation power ($[p/s]/\mu W/cm^2$) values corrected for tissue autofluorescence is described below.

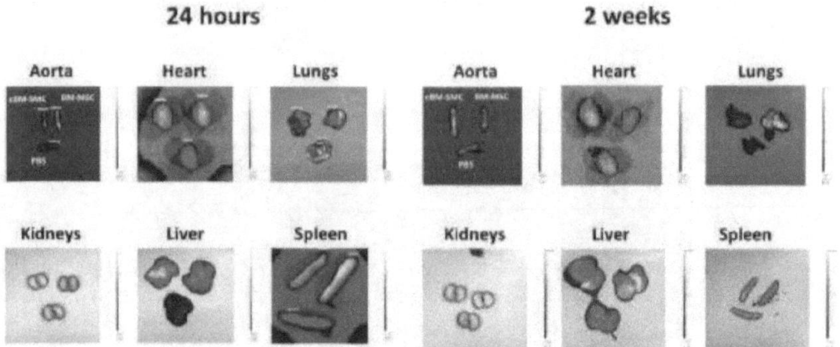

Figure 40. Biodistribution of fluorescently tagged cells in six major organs at 24 hours and 2 weeks as detected by IVIS Spectrum CT

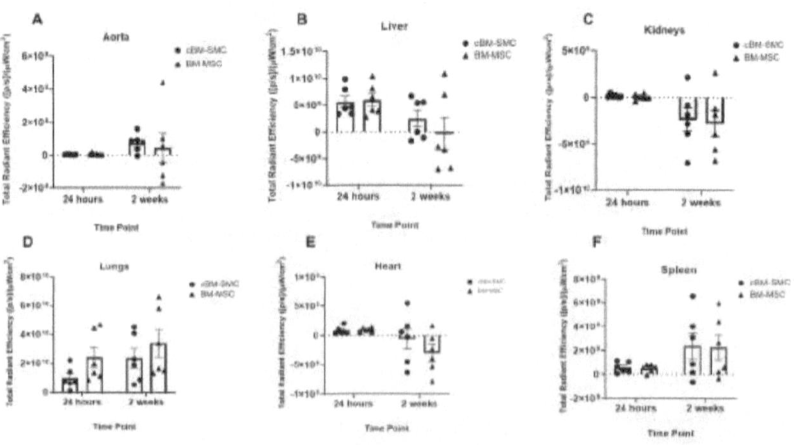

129

5.3.4.1 Aorta: No difference was seen in the distribution of cells in the aorta within the cell types and between the cell types both at 24 hours and 2 weeks **(Figure 41A).**

5.3.4.2 Liver: No difference was seen in the distribution of cells in the liver within the cell types and between the cell types both at 24 hours and 2 weeks **(Figure 41B).**

5.3.4.3 Kidneys: No difference was seen in the distribution of cells in the kidneys within the cell types and between the cell types both at 24 hours and 2 weeks **(Figure 41C).**

5.3.4.4 Lungs: No difference was seen in the distribution of cells in the lungs within the cell types and between the cell types both at 24 hours and 2 weeks **(Figure 41D).**

5.3.4.5 Heart: No difference was seen in the distribution of cells in the heart within the cell types and between the cell types both at 24 hours and 2 weeks **(Figure 41E).**

5.3.4.6 Spleen: No difference was seen in the distribution of cells in the spleen within the cell types and between the cell types both at 24 hours and 2 weeks **(Figure 41F).**

5.3.4.7 **Distribution between the organs at 24 hours and 2 weeks:** The presence of both cBM-SMCs and BM-MSCs was significantly higher in lungs vs all other organs except the liver at 24 hours **(Figure 42A)** whereas at 2 weeks, the distribution of both the cell types was significantly higher in lungs versus all other organs **(Figure 42B)**.

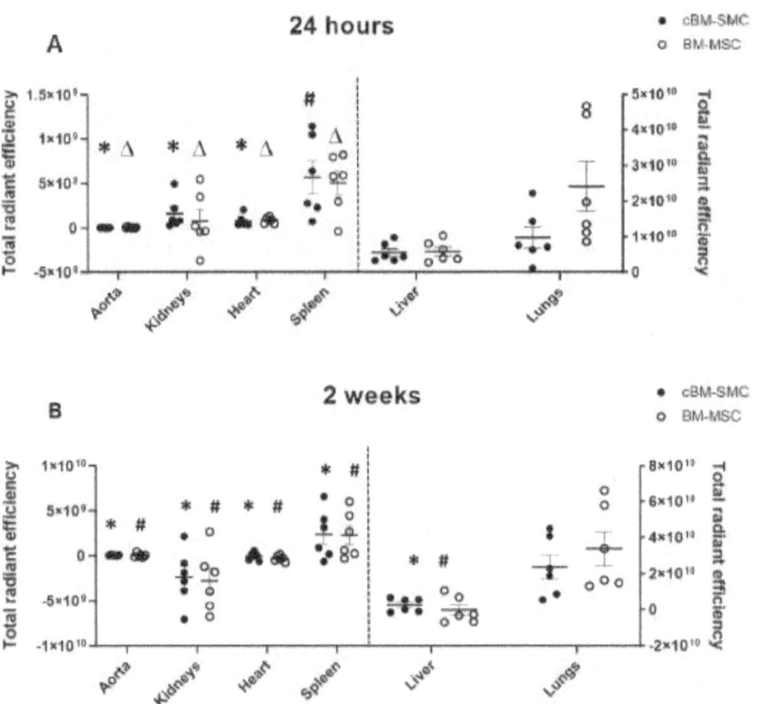

Figure 40. (A) Total fluorescent radiant efficiency comparing all the organs with cBM-SMCs as well as BM-MSCs injections at 24 hours. * represents cBM-SMC's all organs vs Lungs, p < 0.05; # represents cBM-SMC's spleen vs lungs, p = 0.05; Δ represents BM-MSC's all organs vs Lungs, p < 0.001. (B) Total fluorescent radiant efficiency comparing all the organs with cBM-SMCs as well as BM-MSCs injections at 2 weeks. * represents cBM-SMC's all organs vs Lungs, p < 0.003 and # represents BM-MSC's all organs vs Lungs, p < 0.001

5.3.5 C3 complement activation

No difference was seen in the plasma C3 complement protein between cBM-SMC-, BM-SMC- and PBS-injected rats as measured by ELISA at 24 hours as well as 2 weeks of cell injection **(Figure 43 A and B)**.

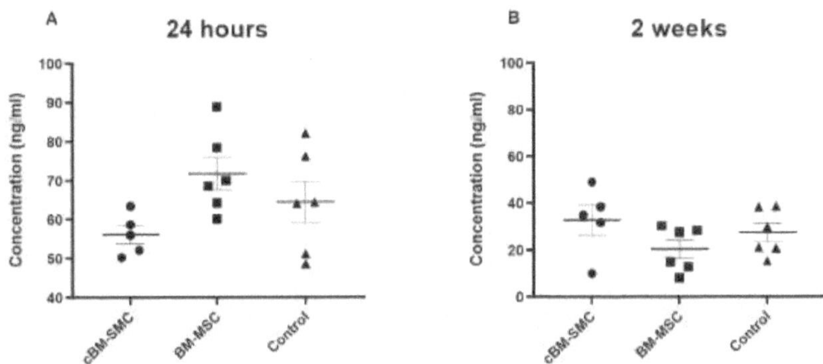

Figure 41. C3 Complement protein concentration (ng/ml) as measured by ELISA at (A) 24 hours and (B) 2 weeks of cell injection

5.3.6 Volumetric assessment of Aorta using Phase Contrast Angiography (PCA) Magnetic Resonance Imaging (MRI)

The results of volumetric assessment of aorta is categorized as below:

5.3.6.1 **Volume changes in aorta with single dose of cell injection:** Percentage change in volume of the aorta at baseline to AAA (B-AAA) versus aorta at baseline to 2 weeks after a single dose treatment (B-2W treatment) was not different for cBM-SMCs while it was significantly lower for BM-MSC and not different ($p = 0.075$) for AAA control or PBS-injected rats **(Figure 44A)**.

5.3.6.2 **Volume changes in aorta with double dose of cell injection:** Percentage change in volume of the aorta at baseline to AAA (B-AAA) versus aorta at baseline to 2 weeks after a single dose treatment (B-2W treatment) was not different for all three groups **(Figure 44B)**.

5.3.6.3 **Effect of dose:** Percentage change in volume of aorta between baseline to 2 weeks after treatment (B-2WT) was significantly higher at single dose versus double doses for cBM-SMCs whereas no difference was seen between the doses for BM-MSC as well as control **(Figure 44C)**.

5.3.6.4 **Effect of time:** Percentage change in volume of aorta between baseline to 2 weeks after treatment (B-2WT) was significantly higher versus baseline to 1 week after treatment (B-1WT) for a single dose of cBM-SMCs whereas no difference was seen for BM-MSCs injected rats as well as AAA Control or PBS injected rats. Percentage change in volume of aorta between baseline to 1 week after treatment (B-1WT) was significantly lower in BM-MSCs versus AAA control **(Figure 44D)**.

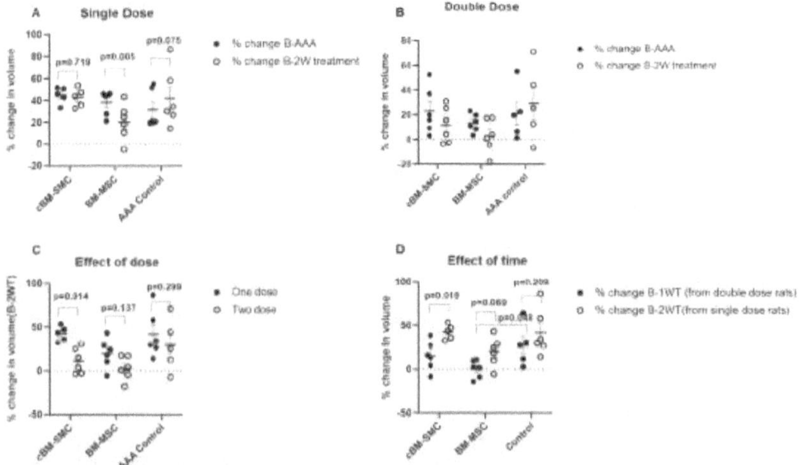

Figure 42: Volume change in aorta subjected to cell treatment. (A) Single dose injection, (B) Double dose injection, (C) Effect of number of cell doses dose on volume change and (D) Effect of time on volume change, shown for a single cell dose

5.3.7   Cytokine Array

The results of the cytokine array presented relative to the untreated AAA

control are summarized in the **Table VI** and **Figures 45 and 46** below.

Table VI: Directionality of cytokines expression changes versus AAA control

Cytokine	Healthy Control	BM-MSC		cBM-SMC	
		One dose	Two doses	One dose	Two doses
IFN-γ	↓	↓	↓	↓	↓
IL-1β	↓	↑	↓	↓	↓
IL-3	=	=	↓	↓	↓
IL-6	↓	↓	↓	↓	↓
IL-17A	↑	↑	↓	↓	↓
TNF-α	↓	↓	↓	↓	↓
MMP-2	↓	↓	↓	↓	↓

MMP-9	↑	↑	↓	↓	↓
Lipocalin-2	↓	↑	↓	↓	↓
MMP-3	↑	↓	↑	↓	↓
Adiponectin	↓	↓	↓	↑	↓
Fetuin A / AHSG	↓	↓	↓	↓	↓
Retinol Binding Protein-4	↓	↓	↓	↓	↓
FGF acidic	=	↓	↓	↑	↓
ICAL-1/CD54	=	=	↓	↓	↑
CXCL-7	↓	↓	↓	↓	↓
NOV/CCN3	↑	↓	↓	↓	↓
IGF-1	↑	↑	↓	=	↑
Fibulin-3	↑	↑	↓	↓	=
CCL11/Eotaxin	↓	↓	↓	↓	↓
Serpin E1/PAI-1	↓	↓	↓	↓	↓
Cystatin C	↓	↓	↓	↓	↓
IGFBP-3	=	↓	↓	↑	↓
Galectin-1	↓	↓	↓	↓	↓
DPPIV/CD26	↓	↓	↓	↓	↓
Osteopontin (OPN)	↓	↓	↓	↓	↓
IGFBP-5	↓	↓	↓	↓	↑
Galectin-3	↓	↓	↓	↓	↓
CCL21/6Ckine	↓	↓	↓	↓	↓
TNFSF12/APO3 ligand	↓	↓	↓	↓	↓
Osteoprotegerin	↓	↓	↓	↓	↓
IGFBP-6	↓	↓	↓	↓	↓
VCAM-1/CD106	↓	↑	↓	↓	↓
Endostatin	↓	↓	↓	↓	↓
Clusterin	↓	↓	↓	↓	↓
CXCL2	↓	↓	↓	↓	↑
EGF	↓	↓	↓	↓	↓
GM-CSF	↑	=	↓	↓	↓
HGF	↑	↑	↓	↓	↑

| PDGF-BB | ↑ | = | ↑ | ↑ | ↑ |
| VEGF | ↓ | ↑ | ↑ | = | = |

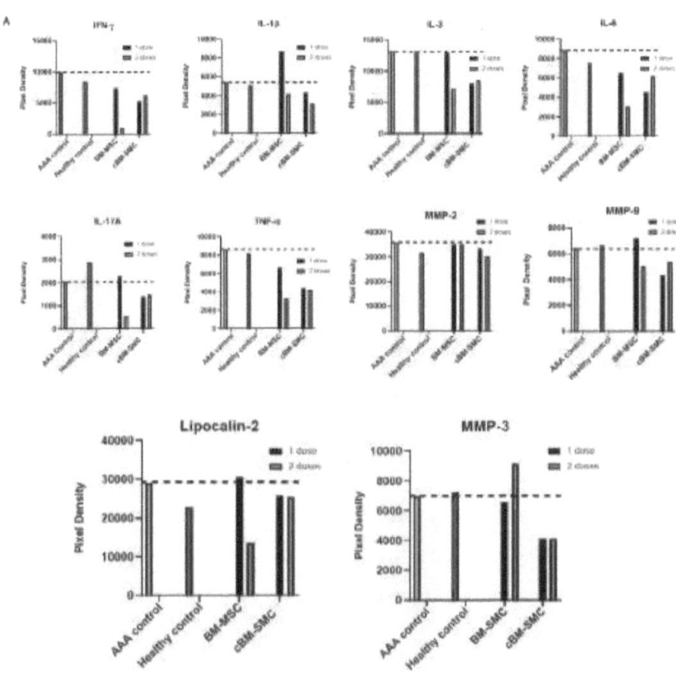

Figure 43: Expression of array of cytokines in the aortal tissue samples. Dotted lines show the level of cytokines in AAA control

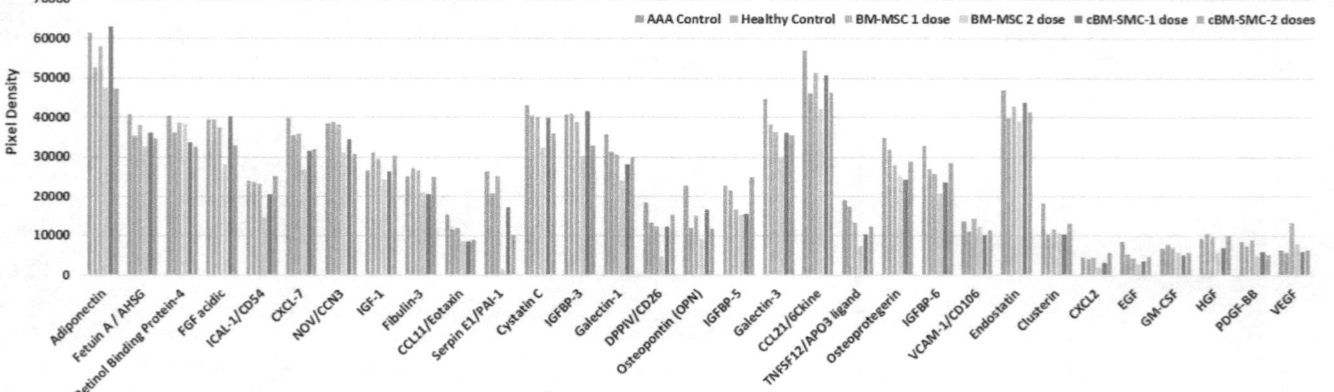

Figure 44: Overall proteome profile of cytokines expressed in aortal tissue samples

5.3.8 Western Blot for elastin homeostasis proteins aorta tissue sample

All results are presented normalized to AAA controls. There were no differences in protein expression between the treatments with either of the cell types for both one and two dose conditions. **(Figure 47)**.

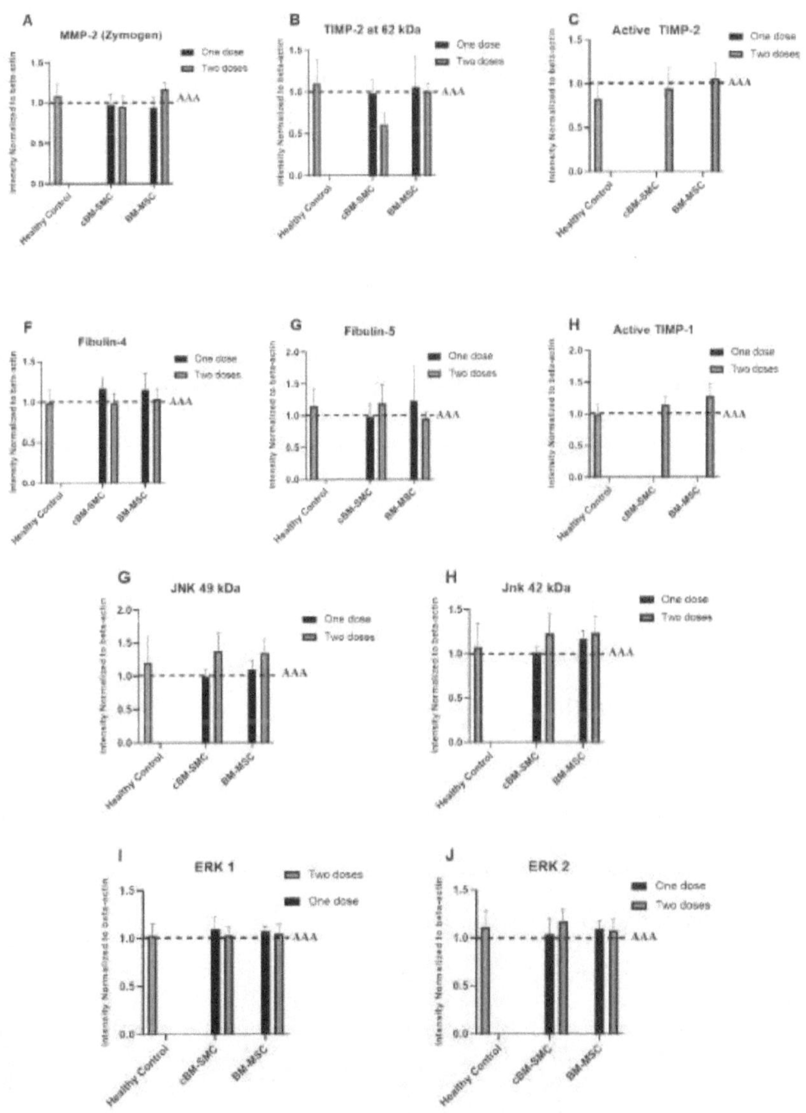

5.4   Discussion

Adult stem cells have been widely used in treatments of cardiovascular disease such as in heart failure, myocardial infarction and ischemic heart disease [171], [272]. Besides their purported ability to home into the tissue site of disease or injury[279], there is also evidence that these stem cells can initiate biological signaling cascades that may work through paracrine mechanisms to regenerate or heal diseased tissues [280]–[282]. In the context of application to cell therapy, there is evidence that mesenchymal stem cells are immune system-privileged and possess anti-inflammatory properties which can reduce the chances of their rejection when allo- or xeno-transplanted [212], [272]. Also, attractiveness is their pluripotency, which allows them to be differentiated into cells of multiple lineages, including cells of the vascular tissues, with prospects to regenerate, repair, and restore function of those tissues [171]. Despite these advantages, factors that limit ready application of these cells to cell therapy include uncertainties as to (a) need for a minimally invasive and mode of cell delivery *in vivo* that ensures cell survival and efficient therapeutic action, b) homing of cells to the target tissue and need for such homing at all, for therapeutic action, (c) long-term engraftment and retention of the cells in target tissues, and in the context of our proposed treatment of AAAs, (d) their ability to effect regenerative elastic matrix repair and reverse the inflammatory and proteolytic pathophysiology in the AAA wall towards slowing AAA growth, and (e) the differences in fate and functional effects of undifferentiated MSCs versus that of their derivatives [283]. Following our generation of well-characterized MSC-derived vascular SMCs, to address these questions, in the this chapter, we describe studies to compare undifferentiated MSCs and MSC-derived SMCs for their natural homing properties, their bio-distribution *in-vivo,* and elastin regenerative benefits and anti-proteolytic/-inflammatory effects if any, in the AAA wall and contribution of these effects to slowing or reversing growth of small AAAs in an elastase injury rat model.

Among all the homing receptors involved in natural homing of BM-MSCs to the disease site, the most common are CXCR4 and CCR3 [284]. Results of studies on CXCR4 and CCR3 gene expression **(Figure 37A and B)** suggests that like undifferentiated BM-MSCs, cBM-SMCs also express these primary homing receptors, implying prospects to home into the diseased site *in vivo*. In fact, our findings suggest that CXCR4 and CCR3 expression is significantly higher in cBM-SMCs vs BM-MSCs regardless of TNF-α priming and priming dose. Although cell priming seemed to have no effect on the expression of both receptors, literature suggests that regardless of the expression of CXCR4, TNF-α might modify the sensitivity of MSCs to SDF-1α (its ligand which is overexpressed in AAA tissue) [284]. This may be achieved by modulating CXCR4 signal transduction without affecting receptor expression itself, through inhibition of the protein kinase C pathway [285]. In contrary to published studies which showed higher CCR3 expression than CXCR4 upon TNF-α stimulation, our results showed significantly lower CCR3 versus CXCR4 gene expression by BM-MSC whereas no such difference was seen in cBM-SMC cultures. However, in congruence with the literature [284], CCR3 protein levels were significantly higher versus CXCR4 for both BM-MSC and cBM-SMCs, as deemed from western blots **(Figure 38)** and immunofluorescence **(Figure 39).** Consistent with published literature [285] immunofluorescence studies showed significantly higher CXCR4 and CCR3 expression on per cell basis by cBM-SMCs versus BM-MSCs likely due to the concomitant expression of the intracellular pool by western blotting. These experiments indicated that (a) cBM-SMCs retain the expression of CCR3 and CXCR4 as the primary homing receptors exhibited by undifferentiated MSCs and hence likely their homing properties, (b) CCR3 expression likely provides a greater homing role/mechanism, and (c) receptor expression itself is unaffected by priming by inflammatory cytokines though their homing to and migration within the AAA wall may be influenced by inhibition of protein kinase C pathway.

Next, we assessed the short term (24 hours) and long-term (2 weeks) bio-distribution of cells *in vivo* upon one time intravenous injection of a cell bolus (2×10^6 cells), specifically their localization in the aorta, liver, kidneys, lungs, heart and spleen). The cell distribution profile **(Figures 41 and 42)** showed that at both assessment time points, and with both BM-MSCs and cBM-SMCs, a dominant fraction of the injected cells were entrapped in lungs. This finding was as we expected since MSC retention in the lungs due to a "pulmonary first pass effect" resulting from their large cell size is well documented [286]. Our results also indicated higher signal associated with presence of BM-MSCs in the lungs compared to the cBM-SMCs, even though the mean difference was not sufficient to show statistical significance, which is likely due to their larger size (~ 10-15 microns for BM-MSCs versus ~ 5 microns for cBM-SMCs). Prior studies have also shown evidence of MSC adhesion to the endothelium of the pulmonary vasculature, which can contribute to the pulmonary first pass effect [286]. Ruster et.al showed that P-selectin and a counter ligand can contribute to adhesion and extravasation of MSCs in the lungs [287]. While this might also be a possibility with our cBM-SMCs which as BM-MSC derivatives share many of their characteristics, further investigation is required to determine the factors that contribute to their localization in the lungs as well as to obtain the statistical difference. We also found reduced distribution of BM-MSCs in the liver, heart and kidneys at 2 weeks versus 24 hours a result that was mimicked by cBM-SMCs although the mean difference was not sufficient to show statistical significant. Differently, both the cell types showed near significant (p = 0.06) time-dependent increases in localization in the spleen. These results evoke published work that have shown rapid interaction of transplanted stem cells with the cells of the immune system through circulating leukocytes or those in the skin, spleen and lymph nodes [288]. The entrapment of transplanted cells in the spleen is also suggested to be a potential mechanism of the immune suppressive effects of MSCs. Indeed, studies have shown that shifts in ratio of regulatory T-cells to cytotoxic CD8+ T- cells and also the polarization of TH1 cells to a cytokine profile-altered TH2 phenotype in splenocytes reduces antibody formation and T-cell responses against the transplanted allogeneic MSCs, hence failing to identify them [288], [289]. Some studies also suggest that entrapment of MSCs in the spleen and resulting T cell responses to be the potential route of MSC clearance however the existence of physiological clearance pathways for transplanted MSCs still remain unelucidated. No activation of C3 complement **(Figure 43)** relative to the PBS injected control animals provides further corroboration that our injected cells do not trigger an immune response, although their ability to lower basal expression of the C3 complement to levels in healthy animals was not assessed.

The volumetric assessment of aorta pre and post cell injection using MRI **(Figure 44)** shows that while injection of a single dose of BM-MSCs caused a significant active reduction in volume of the AAA segment, cBM-SMCs at least prevented an increase in segment volume. When the dose frequency was increased (2 versus 1 dose), we observed a trend of decreasing AAA segment volume although the mean difference was not sufficient to be statistically significant, which is likely due to small sample size and animal to animal variability. However, power analysis of our data predicts that with sample size of 36 animals per group, the statistical significance will be evident. Differently, when comparing the effect of repeat dosing, a double dose seems to be more effective for both cell types, which is also explained by the results of effect of time (2 weeks versus 1 week post-injection) which shows that without a repeat dose of cells 1 week after the first, the volume of aorta tends to increase over the 2 week assessment.

The overall effect of changes in the volume of aorta was also supported by the results of the cytokine array, which showed the expression of a large number of documented inflammatory cytokines (**Table VII** below) to be reduced upon cell treatment. **Table VII** below shows the role and directionality of change in AAA of various cytokines that were detected in the cell treated aortal samples.

Table VII: Role and directionality of change of cytokine expression in AAA

Cytokine	Role in AAA	Directionality of Change in AAA	References
IFN-γ	Induces cathepsin S from vascular SMCs, inhibits collagen production, promotes inflammation by stimulating T and B lymphocytes, macrophages, endothelial cells fibroblasts	Upregulated	[290], [291]
IL-1β	Initiate the inflammatory cascade pertinent to AAA, trigger expression of many other cytokines, cyclic expression of itself, co-localization with AAA SMCs	Upregulated	[292]

IL-6	Inflammatory cell migration and infiltration, minor role in tissue disruption during inflammation, ECM remodeling, expression of tissue degrading proteases, SMC apoptosis	Upregulated	[293]
IL-17A	Modulates systemic and vascular inflammation by stimulating IFN-γ production, increases vascular reactive oxygen species and vascular leukocyte infiltration, induces production of other cytokines in the vascular wall, increases superoxide production	Upregulated	[294]
TNF-α	Activation and recruitment of immune cells to the sites of inflammation, secretion of proinflammatory cytokines and MMPs, initiation of SMC and fibroblast apoptosis	Upregulated	[295]
MMP-2	Elastolysis and matrix remodeling	Upregulated	[296]
MMP-9	Elastolysis and matrix remodeling	Upregulated	[296]
Lipocalin-2	Leukocyte recruitment, MMP-9 stability and activation, potential role in apoptosis of VSMCs	Upregulated	[297]
MMP-3	Weakens aorta wall, adds up proteolysis by activating other latent MMPs	Upregulated	[298]

We further assessed elastin homeostasis in cell treated aorta to provide the initial evidence of elastin regenerative benefit **(Figure 47)**. Even though we did not see statistical significance in the protein expression level of elastin homeostasis proteins like MMPs (proteolytic enzymes), Fibulin – 4 and 5 (elastin fiber assembly) between the cell types or between one or two dosings for each cell type, the absence of active MMP-2 and MMP-9 as well as presence of active TIMP-1 and TIMP-2 upon 2 doses of cell treatment can be deemed a positive outcome in terms of elastin preservation. This was further supported by the visual representation of elastin fibers using modified HART staining **(Figure 48)** which clearly shows thick, matured and continuous fibers in cBM-SMCs treated aorta whereas fragmented and thinner fibers in BM-MSCs treated aorta or the AAA control. We did not see any statistical difference in JNK or ERK 1/2 expression upon cell treatment likely because these pathways are implicated more in larger aneurysms and in this body of work we have focused on smaller aneurysms.

Overall, our results suggests that cBM-SMCs like BM-MSCs have potential to home in to the AAA site, cBM-SMCs retain in AAA site for longer time period compared to BM-MSCs, cell treatment potentially attenuates overall inflammation and regresses aneurysm growth even more efficiently with 2 doses of cell injection.

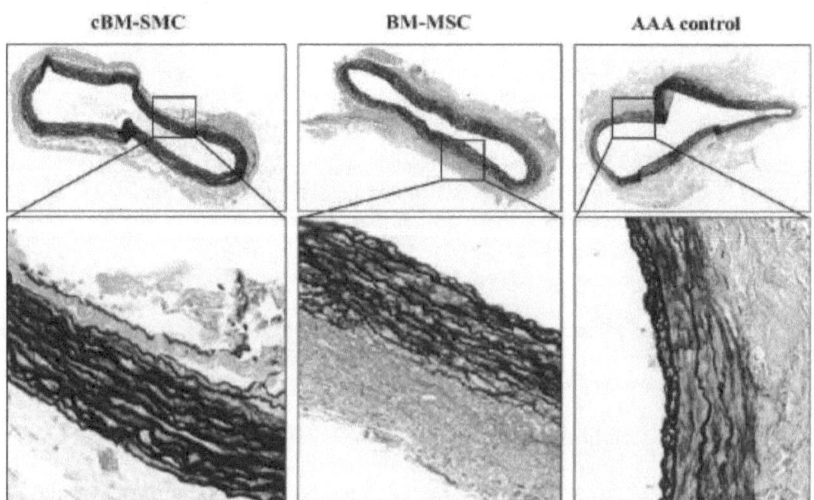

Figure 46: Modified hart stained aorta tissue section after cell treatment

Chapter VI

CONCLUSIONS AND FUTURE DIRECTIONS

6.1 Overall Conclusions

In this body of work, we explored the utility of BM-MSCs and their smooth muscle cell derivatives of select phenotypes as an approach for regenerating and repairing extracellular matrix in the aorta wall towards stabilizing small AAAs and growth. Since, vascular elastic matrix is synthesized in a developmental tissue milieu rich in stem cells and progenitor cells, in our previous body of work, we successfully confirmed a hypothesis that stem cell derived smooth muscle cell-like cells (SMLCs) of specific phenotypes would exhibit superior elastogenicity than do healthy and diseased adult vascular SMCs and in addition demonstrated that the derived cells provide pro-elastogenic and anti-proteolytic stimuli to diseased cells. However, for cell therapy applications, a large inoculate of cells, which mandates extensive, long-term propagation in culture. For reliable benefits to tissue repair, phenotypic stability of the derived cells and their maintenance of their superior elastin regenerative properties in a pathophysiology-mimicking collagenous AAA milieu not conducive to elastogenesis, are vitally important. Besides clarifying this, this study contributes vitally to providing an understanding of the fate of the derived cells in an *in vivo* rat model of small AAAs, their homing properties relative to undifferentiated BM-MSCs and has generated evidence of their benefits to stabilizing small AAAs against growth. Our primary findings were:

(1)   The BM-MSCs derived BM-SMCs better retained their differentiated phenotype upon continued provision of the differentiation substrate and growth factor conditions during propagation. The differentiated cells propagated under such conditions were designated as cBM-SMCs. We also found that these cells were of early intermediate phenotype as shown by robust expression of alpha smooth muscle actin (ACTA-2), an early stage marker but not Myosin Heavy Chain (MYH 11), a late stage marker. We found that cBM-SMCs were also more elastogenic as suggested by the expression of LOX, Fibulin-4 and Fibulin-5, desmosine as well as the TEM images which showed robust elastic fibers in cBM-SMCs.

(2)   In a simulated 3-D collagenous tissue milieu evocative of the de-elasticized aorta wall, cBM-SMCs retained their SMC phenotype and superior elastogenicity and anti-proteolytic activity. We found significantly higher total matrix elastin, which was corroborated by VVG staining of the constructs. With VVG staining we saw robust, matured and thick elastin fibers in constructs containing standalone cBM-SMCs or co-culture of cBM-SMCs with EaRASMCs suggesting that cBM-SMCs in addition to generating elastin, also provide elastogenic stimulus to cultured aneurysmal smooth muscle cells (EaRASMCs) from our rat model.

(3)   We found that cBM-SMCs as per our hypothesis, cBM-SMCs also possessed the homing ability like BM-MSCs, with involvement of the same CCR3 and CXCR4

receptors. In fact, we saw significantly higher expression of both CXCR4 and CCR3 in cBM-SMCs vs BM-MSCs. We also, saw that priming with TNF-α did not make significant difference in expression of homing receptors and among the two receptors, CCR3 is expressed more compared to CXCR4. Thus, our results suggest that CCR3 might be the primary homing receptor driving the homing of cBM-SMCs to the AAA site.

(4)   Our *in vivo* studies indicated infused cells of both types to primarily engraft in the lungs to be retained for at least 2 weeks, although cell presence in the aorta was also noted. While no differences in BM-MSC presence in the aneurysmal aorta segment were noted between 24 hours and 2 weeks, significantly higher number of cBM-SMCs were seen in the aneurysmal aorta at the 2 week time point, suggesting prolonged homing and retention of cells in the AAA vessel segment. Similarly, the higher expression of both cell types in the spleen at 2 weeks suggests the clearance of cells via spleen as documented in literature. Our studies also indicated lack of immune complement C3 activation by the cell types *in vivo*, vital to safe application for cell therapy.

(5)   Our results provide strong evidence as to the ability of the infused cells (both BM-MSC and cBM-SMCs) to downregulate expression of several inflammatory and pro-apoptotic cytokines that are upregulated in the AAA wall, contributing to accelerated elastic matrix breakdown and suppression of elastic fiber neoassembly, repair and crosslinking. Our results also indicated signficantly improved elastic matrix in the AAA wall upon treatment with the cBM-SMCs but not the BM-MSCs or saline treatment; modified HART stained aortal tissue sections which showed thick and matured fibers on cBM-SMCs treated aorta

whereas the fibers were thinner and fragmented in the BM-MSCs treated and PBS treated AAA control. The results suggest effectiveness of cBM-SMCs in reversing AAA pathophysiology.

(6)   Volumetric assessment of the aneurysmal aorta segment using MRI/PCA showed that a single dose of cBM-SMCs did not allow aorta to grow bigger in volume whereas with double dose the aortal volume was considerably reduced at 2 weeks.

Thus, the overall initial evidence shows the prospective utility of cBM-SMCs as potential cell source for cell therapy to reverse pathophysiology of matrix degradative conditions like AAAs by imparting elastogenic impetus to the diseased cells, reducing inflammation.

6.2   Limitations of the study

Although the results of this study were in accordance with our hypothesis, there were some limitations which are listed below:

(1)   Our study investigated differential expression of homing receptors by our BM-MSCs and cBM-SMCs but did not specifically examine the mechanisms of homing.

(2)   The small sample size in the experimental groups used in the *in vivo* study was insufficient to observe statistical significance of outcomes for several studied parameters.

(3)   For assessment of cell biodistribution we did not perform a longitudinal study. Such a study would provide vital information of temporal changes in the

migration of cells to different organs and their retention in situ over the period of 2 weeks.

(4)   Some of the background subtracted total radiant efficiency values for organs like kidneys and liver were negative. We assume this is due to very minimal presence of tagged cells associated fluorescence and very high inherent autofluorescence of the organs.

(5)   In 1 out of 6 BM-MSC injected rats for each one dose and 2 dose experiments we saw tumor formation in the kidneys. At this time, we are unclear if this is a direct BM-MSC-generated effect and how the diseased milieu influenced the matrix regenerative outcomes in the AAA.

6.3   Future Recommendations

Based on our findings in this study, I propose the following recommendations for future work:

(1)   Investigate the mechanism(s) underlying homing of cBM-SMCs from circulation to the AAA wall and engineer or prime the cells to enhance their homing potential. Treatment with vasodilators can also help to reduce or overcome the pulmonary first pass effect.

(2)   Enhance rigor of the in vivo assessments and ensure statistical significance of differences in key parameters between groups through study of much larger numbers of replicate animals/group. We have performed power analysis of our current data to predict the animal numbers that would be required to limit animal to animal variability and ensure statistical significance between experimental

groups. Similarly, in a future study, the treatment period can be extended well beyond 2 weeks, which will provide the opportunity to test the efficacy of cell therapy with greater rigor.

(3) Utilize advanced MRI techniques to perform a non-invasive longitudinal study of matrix changes in the AAA wall over time rather than performing end point analysis for each animal at each time point. Also, for ex-vivo imaging, use large number of controls so that the controls can be tightened which might reduce the negative value of radiant efficiency. As well as take necessary precaution like pat drying the tissue uniformly to avoid high background fluorescence.

(4) Investigate the matrix regenerative and reparative potential of cBM-SMCs in larger, critically-sized AAAs.

(5) Explore utility of cBM-SMCs for correcting lung elastinopathies like COPD or emphysema, which will leverage their entrapment in the pulmonary vasculature.

(6) Assess the homing properties of the cells and determine the relative contributions of cell localization in the aneurysmal aorta and in the lungs to the pro-matrix regenerative benefits through the necessary and sufficient paracrine mechanisms.

(7) Also assess if the knowledge of the necessary and sufficient secreted factors can be leveraged for delivery from non-cellular vehicles like exosomes, nanoparticles, scaffolds, etc.

REFERENCES

[1]   H. Kuivaniemi, E. J. Ryer, J. R. Elmore, and G. Tromp, "Understanding the pathogenesis of abdominal aortic aneurysms," *Expert Rev. Cardiovasc. Ther.*, vol. 13, no. 9, pp. 975–987, Sep. 2015, doi: 10.1586/14779072.2015.1074861.

[2]   A. Daugherty and L. A. Cassis, "Mechanisms of abdominal aortic aneurysm formation.," *Curr. Atheroscler. Rep.*, vol. 4, no. 3, pp. 222–227, 2002, doi: 10.1007/s11883-002-0023-5.

[3]   B. Sivaraman, C. A. Bashur, and A. Ramamurthi, "Advances in biomimetic regeneration of elastic matrix structures," *Drug Deliv. Transl. Res.*, vol. 2, no. 5, pp. 323–350, 2012, doi: 10.1007/s13346-012-0070-6.

[4]   S. M. Mithieux and A. S. Weiss, "Elastin," *Adv. Protein Chem.*, vol. 70, pp. 437–461, 2005, doi: 10.1016/S0065-3233(05)70013-9.

[5]   G. Swaminathan, I. Stoilov, T. Broekelmann, R. Mecham, and A. Ramamurthi, "Phenotype-based selection of bone marrow mesenchymal stem cell-derived smooth muscle cells for elastic matrix regenerative repair in abdominal aortic aneurysms," *J. Tissue Eng. Regen. Med.*, vol. 12, no. 1, pp. e60–e70, 2018, doi: 10.1002/term.2349.

[6]   G. Swaminathan, V. S. Gadepalli, I. Stoilov, R. P. Mecham, R. R. Rao, and A. Ramamurthi, "Pro-elastogenic effects of bone marrow mesenchymal stem cell-derived smooth muscle cells on cultured aneurysmal smooth muscle cells," *J. Tissue Eng. Regen. Med.*, vol. 11, no. 3, pp. 679–693, 2017, doi: 10.1002/term.1964.

[7]   Z. S. Alyami and M. M. Alotaibi, "Abdominal Aortic Aneurysm : A

        Comprehensive Review = تمدد الشريان الأبهري البطني: دراسة شاملة," *Al-Azhar Med.*

        J., vol. 45, no. 3, pp. 559–570, 2017, doi: 10.12816/0033123.

[8]   J. Chuen and M. Theivendran, "Abdominal aortic aneurysm: An update," *Aust.*

        J. Gen. Pract., vol. 47, no. 5, pp. 252–256, 2018, doi: 10.31128/AFP-09-17-

        4340.

[9]   J. Golledge and P. E. Norman, "Current status of medical management for

        abdominal aortic aneurysm," *Atherosclerosis*, vol. 217, no. 1, pp. 57–63, Jul.

        2011, doi: 10.1016/j.atherosclerosis.2011.03.006.

[10]   B. T. Baxter, M. C. Terrin, and R. L. Dalman, "Medical management of small

        abdominal aortic aneurysms," *Circulation*, vol. 117, no. 14, pp. 1883–9, 2008,

        doi: 10.1161/CIRCULATIONAHA.107.735274.

[11]   W. P. Daley, S. B. Peters, and M. Larsen, "Extracellular matrix dynamics in

        development and regenerative medicine," *Journal of Cell Science*. 2008, doi:

        10.1242/jcs.006064.

[12]   H. Jarvelainen, A. Sainio, M. Koulu, T. N. Wight, and R. Pennttinen,

        "Extracellular matrix molecules: Potential Targets in Pharmacotherapy,"

        Pharmacol. Rev., vol. 61, no. 2, pp. 198–223, 2009, doi:

        10.1124/pr.109.001289.

[13]   C. Frantz, K. M. Stewart, and V. M. Weaver, "The extracellular matrix at a

        glance," *Journal of Cell Science*. 2010, doi: 10.1242/jcs.023820.

[14]   F. H. Silver, I. Horvath, and D. J. Foran, "Viscoelasticity of the vessel wall:

The role of collagen and elastic fibers," *Critical Reviews in Biomedical Engineering*. 2001, doi: 10.1615/critrevbiomedeng.v29.i3.10.

[15]   P. Berillis, "The Role of Collagen in the Aorta's Structure," *Open Circ. Vasc. J.*, 2013, doi: 10.2174/1877382601306010001.

[16]   B. Yue, "Biology of Extracellular Matrix: An Overview," *J. Glycoma*, vol. 23, pp. S20–S23, 2015, doi: 10.1097/IJG.0000000000000108.Biology.

[17]   M. Durbeej, "Laminins," *Cell and Tissue Research*. 2010, doi: 10.1007/s00441-009-0838-2.

[18]   J. E. Schwarzbauer and D. W. DeSimone, "Fibronectins, their fibrillogenesis, and in vivo functions," *Cold Spring Harbor Perspectives in Biology*. 2011, doi: 10.1101/cshperspect.a005041.

[19]   R. V Iozzo and L. Schaefer, "Proteoglycan form and function: A comprehensive nomenclature of proteoglycans," *Matrix Biol.*, vol. 42, pp. 11–55, 2015, doi: 10.1016/j.matbio.2015.02.003.Proteoglycan.

[20]   L. Schaefer and R. M. Schaefer, "Proteoglycans : from structural compounds to signaling molecules," *Cell Tissue Res.*, vol. 339, pp. 237–246, 2010, doi: 10.1007/s00441-009-0821-y.

[21]   S. Mizumoto, S. Ikegawa, and K. Sugahara, "Human Genetic Disorders Caused by Mutations in Genes Encoding Biosynthetic Enzymes for," *J. Biol. Chem.*, vol. 288, no. 16, pp. 10953–10961, 2013, doi: 10.1074/jbc.R112.437038.

[22]   S. Liliana and R. V. Iozzo, "Biological Functions of the Small Leucine-rich Proteoglycans : From Genetics to Signal Transduction *," *J. Biol. Chem.*, vol.

283, no. 31, pp. 21305–21309, 2008, doi: 10.1074/jbc.R800020200.

[23]   M. Barczyk, S. Carracedo, and D. Gullberg, "Integrins," *Cell Tissue Res.*, vol. 339, pp. 269–280, 2010, doi: 10.1007/s00441-009-0834-6.

[24]   H. Wolfenson, I. Lavelin, and B. Geiger, "Dynamic Regulation of the Structure and Functions of Integrin Adhesions," *Dev Cell*, vol. 24, no. 5, pp. 447–58, 2013, doi: 10.1016/j.devcel.2013.02.012.Dynamic.

[25]   B. Geiger and K. M. Yamada, "Molecular Architecture and Function of Matrix Adhesions," *Cold Spring Harb. Perspect. Biol.*, vol. 3, pp. 1–21, 2011.

[26]   P. Lu, K. Takai, V. M. Weaver, and Z. Werb, "Extracellular Matrix Degradation and Remodeling in Development and Disease," *Cold Spring Harb. Perspect. Biol.*, vol. 3, pp. 1–24, 2011.

[27]   P. A. Jones, T. Scott-Burden, and W. Gevers, "Glycoprotein , elastin , and collagen secretion by rat smooth muscle cells," *Cell Biol.*, vol. 76, no. 1, pp. 353–357, 1979, doi: 10.1073/pnas.76.1.353.

[28]   Gh. C. Sephel and J. M. Davidson, "Elastin Production in Human Skin Fibroblast Cultures and Its Decline with Age," *J. Investgative Dermatology*, vol. 86, no. 3, pp. 279–285, 1985, doi: 10.1111/1523-1747.ep12285424.

[29]   J. Uitto, A. M. Christiano, V. Kahari, M. M. Bashir, and J. Rosenbloomt, "Molecular biology and pathology of human elastin," *Biochem. Soc. Transa*, vol. 19, pp. 824–829, 1989.

[30]   A. Hinek, R. P. Mecham, F. Keeley, and M. Rabinovitch, "Impaired elastin fiber assembly related to reduced 67-kD elastin-binding protein in fetal lamb

ductus arteriosus and in cultured aortic smooth muscle cells treated with chondroitin sulfate," *J. Clin. Invest.*, vol. 88, no. 6, pp. 2083–2094, 1991, doi: 10.1172/JCI115538.

[31]   L. E. Grosso and R. P. Mecham, "In vitro processing of tropoelastin: investigation of a possible transport function associated with the carboxy-terminal domain.," *Biochem. Biophys. Res. Commun.*, vol. 153, no. 2, pp. 545–551, Jun. 1988, doi: 10.1016/s0006-291x(88)81129-x.

[32]   A. Hinek, F. W. Keeley, and J. Callahan, "Recycling of the 67-kDa elastin binding protein in arterial myocytes is imperative for secretion of tropoelastin.," *Exp. Cell Res.*, vol. 220, no. 2, pp. 312–324, Oct. 1995, doi: 10.1006/excr.1995.1321.

[33]   B. S. M. Mithieux and A. S. Weiss, "Elastin," *Adv. Protein Chem.*, vol. 70, no. 4, pp. 437–461, 2006, doi: 10.1016/S0065-3233(04)70013-3.

[34]   S. Privitera, C. A. Prody, J. W. Callahan, and A. Hinek, "The 67-kDa Enzymatically Inactive Alternatively Spliced Variant of ˋ -Galactosidase Is Identical to the Elastin / Laminin-binding Protein *," vol. 273, no. 11, pp. 6319–6326, 1998.

[35]   X. Liu *et al.*, "Elastic fiber homeostasis requires lysyl oxidase-like 1 protein.," *Nat. Genet.*, vol. 36, no. 2, pp. 178–182, Feb. 2004, doi: 10.1038/ng1297.

[36]   E. Noblesse *et al.*, "Lysyl oxidase-like and lysyl oxidase are present in the dermis and epidermis of a skin equivalent and in human skin and are associated to elastic fibers.," *J. Invest. Dermatol.*, vol. 122, no. 3, pp. 621–630, Mar. 2004, doi: 10.1111/j.0022-202X.2004.22330.x.

[37]   H. M. Kagan and K. A. Sullivan, "Lysyl oxidase: preparation and role in elastin biosynthesis.," *Methods Enzymol.*, vol. 82 Pt A, pp. 637–650, 1982, doi: 10.1016/0076-6879(82)82092-2.

[38]   P. Brown-Augsburger, C. Tisdale, T. Broekelmann, C. Sloan, and R. P. Mecham, "Identification of an elastin cross-linking domain that joins three peptide chains. Possible role in nucleated assembly.," *J. Biol. Chem.*, vol. 270, no. 30, pp. 17778–17783, Jul. 1995, doi: 10.1074/jbc.270.30.17778.

[39]   A. W. Clarke, S. G. Wise, S. A. Cain, C. M. Kielty, and A. S. Weiss, "Coacervation Is Promoted by Molecular Interactions between the PF2 Segment of Fibrillin-1 and the Domain 4 Region of Tropoelastin †," *Biochemistry*, vol. 44, no. 30, pp. 10271–10281, 2006, doi: 10.1021/bi050530d.

[40]   C. M. K. M. J. S. and C. A. Shuttleworth, "Elastic Fibres," *J. Cell Sci.*, vol. 115, no. 14, pp. 2817–2828, 2002.

[41]   L. Debelle and A. J. Alix, "The structures of elastins and their function.," *Biochimie*, vol. 81, no. 10, pp. 981–994, Oct. 1999, doi: 10.1016/s0300-9084(99)00221-7.

[42]   J. A. Eble and S. Niland, "The extracellular matrix of blood vessels.," *Curr. Pharm. Des.*, vol. 15, no. 12, pp. 1385–1400, 2009, doi: 10.2174/138161209787846757.

[43]   L. B. Sandberg, D. Ph, N. T. Soskel, and T. B. Wolt, "Structure of the Elastic Fiber : An Overview," no. 113, 1982, doi: 10.1038/jid.1982.24.

[44]   C. Frantz, K. M. Stewart, and V. M. Weaver, "The extracellular matrix at a

glance," *J. Cell Sci.*, vol. 123, no. 24, pp. 4195–4200, Dec. 2010, doi: 10.1242/jcs.023820.

[45] J. E. Wagenseil and R. P. Mecham, "Vascular extracellular matrix and arterial mechanics.," *Physiol. Rev.*, vol. 89, no. 3, pp. 957–989, Jul. 2009, doi: 10.1152/physrev.00041.2008.

[46] I. Pasquali-Ronchetti and M. Baccarani-Contri, "Elastic fiber during development and aging.," *Microsc. Res. Tech.*, vol. 38, no. 4, pp. 428–435, Aug. 1997, doi: 10.1002/(SICI)1097-0029(19970815)38:4<428::AID-JEMT10>3.0.CO;2-L.

[47] M. A. Dubick, R. B. Rucker, and L. Lollinl, "Elastin Turnover in Murine Lung after Repeated Ozone Exposure Ozone (0 ,) is an irritant gas that is ubiquitious in many urban atmospheres . It has been observed that up to 90 % of oxidant smog , such as that found in Southern Cali- fornia in the dayti," *Toxicol. Appl. Pharmacol.*, vol. 58, pp. 203–210, 1981.

[48] K. Suyama and F. Nakamura, "Isolation and Characterization of New Crosslinking Amino Acid ' Allodesmosine' from Hydrolysate of Elastin," *Biochem. Biophys. Res. Commun.*, vol. 170, no. 2, pp. 713–718, 1990.

[49] R. Visse and H. Nagase, "Matrix Metalloproteinases and Tissue Inhibitors of Metalloproteinases," *Circ. Res.*, vol. 92, pp. 827–839, 2003, doi: 10.1161/01.RES.0000070112.80711.3D.

[50] J. H. N. Lindeman, "The pathophysiologic basis of abdominal aortic aneurysm progression : a critical appraisal," *Expert Rev. Cardiovasc. Ther.*, vol. 13, no. 7, pp. 839–851, 2015, doi: 10.1586/14779072.2015.1052408.

[51] X. Wang and R. A. Khalil, "Matrix Metalloproteinases, Vascular Remodeling, and Vascualar Disease," *Advvanced Pharmacol.*, vol. 81, pp. 241–330, 2018, doi: 10.1016/bs.alpha.2017.08.002.

[52] W. Mingyi *et al.*, "Matrix Metalloproteinase 2 Activation of Transforming Growth Factor-β1 (TGF-β1) and TGF-β1–Type II Receptor Signaling Within the Aged Arterial Wall," *Arterioscler. Thromb. Vasc. Biol.*, vol. 26, no. 7, pp. 1503–1509, Jul. 2006, doi: 10.1161/01.ATV.0000225777.58488.f2.

[53] H. Nagase, R. Visse, and G. Murphy, "Structure and function of matrix metalloproteinases and TIMPs.," *Cardiovasc. Res.*, vol. 69, no. 3, pp. 562–573, Feb. 2006, doi: 10.1016/j.cardiores.2005.12.002.

[54] M. D. Sternlicht and Z. Werb, "How matrix metalloproteinases regulate cell behavior.," *Annu. Rev. Cell Dev. Biol.*, vol. 17, pp. 463–516, 2001, doi: 10.1146/annurev.cellbio.17.1.463.

[55] H. Nagase and J. F. J. Woessner, "Matrix metalloproteinases.," *J. Biol. Chem.*, vol. 274, no. 31, pp. 21491–21494, Jul. 1999, doi: 10.1074/jbc.274.31.21491.

[56] S. F. G., "Matrix Metalloproteinases," *Circ. Res.*, vol. 90, no. 5, pp. 520–530, Mar. 2002, doi: 10.1161/01.RES.0000013290.12884.A3.

[57] S. Sjoberg and S. Guo-Ping, "Cysteine Protease Cathepsins in Atherosclerosis and Abdominal Aortic Aneurysm," *Clin Rev Bone Min. Metab.*, vol. 9, no. 2, pp. 138–147, 2012, doi: 10.1007/s12018-011-9098-2.Cysteine.

[58] J. Liu *et al.*, "Cathepsin L expression and regulation in human abdominal aortic aneurysm, atherosclerosis, and vascular cells.," *Atherosclerosis*, vol. 184, pp.

302–311, 2006, doi: 10.1016/j.atherosclerosis.2005.05.012.

[59]   G. P. Shi *et al.*, "Cystatin C deficiency in human atherosclerosis and aortic aneurysms.," *J. Clin. Invest.*, vol. 104, no. 9, pp. 1191–1197, Nov. 1999, doi: 10.1172/JCI7709.

[60]   H. Abdul-Hussien *et al.*, "Collagen degradation in the abdominal aneurysm: a conspiracy of matrix metalloproteinase and cysteine collagenases.," *Am. J. Pathol.*, vol. 170, no. 3, pp. 809–817, Mar. 2007, doi: 10.2353/ajpath.2007.060522.

[61]   G. K. Sukhova, G. P. Shi, D. I. Simon, H. A. Chapman, and P. Libby, "Expression of the elastolytic cathepsins S and K in human atheroma and regulation of their production in smooth muscle cells.," *J. Clin. Invest.*, vol. 102, no. 3, pp. 576–583, Aug. 1998, doi: 10.1172/JCI181.

[62]   S. J. Van Vickle-Chavez *et al.*, "Temporal changes in mouse aortic wall gene expression during the development of elastase-induced abdominal aortic aneurysms.," *J. Vasc. Surg.*, vol. 43, no. 5, pp. 1010–1020, May 2006, doi: 10.1016/j.jvs.2006.01.004.

[63]   M. B. Pagano *et al.*, "Critical role of dipeptidyl peptidase I in neutrophil recruitment during the development of experimental abdominal aortic aneurysms.," *Proc. Natl. Acad. Sci. U. S. A.*, vol. 104, no. 8, pp. 2855–2860, Feb. 2007, doi: 10.1073/pnas.0606091104.

[64]   Z. Urbán and C. D. Boyd, "Elastic-Fiber Pathologies: Primary Defects in Assembly—and Secondary Disorders in Transport and Delivery," *Am. J. Hum. Genet.*, vol. 67, no. 1, pp. 4–7, Jul. 2002, doi: 10.1086/302987.

[65]   Z. Urbán *et al.*, "Isolated supravalvular aortic stenosis: functional

haploinsufficiency of the elastin gene as a result of nonsense-mediated

decay.," *Hum. Genet.*, vol. 106, no. 6, pp. 577–588, Jun. 2000, doi:

10.1007/s004390000285.

[66]   M. C. Zhang, L. He, M. Giro, S. L. Yong, G. E. Tiller, and J. M. Davidson,

"Cutis laxa arising from frameshift mutations in exon 30 of the elastin gene

(ELN).," *J. Biol. Chem.*, vol. 274, no. 2, pp. 981–986, Jan. 1999, doi:

10.1074/jbc.274.2.981.

[67]   M. Tassabehji *et al.*, "An elastin gene mutation producing abnormal

tropoelastin and abnormal elastic fibres in a patient with autosomal dominant

cutis laxa.," *Hum. Mol. Genet.*, vol. 7, no. 6, pp. 1021–1028, Jun. 1998, doi:

10.1093/hmg/7.6.1021.

[68]   F. Ramirez, "Fibrill1n mutations in Marfan syndrome and related phenotypes.,"

Curr. Opin. Genet. Dev., vol. 6, no. 3, pp. 309–315, Jun. 1996, doi:

10.1016/s0959-437x(96)80007-4.

[69]   H. C. Dietz and R. E. Pyeritz, "Mutations in the human gene for fibrillin-1

(FBN1) in the Marfan syndrome and related disorders.," *Hum. Mol. Genet.*,

vol. 4 Spec No, pp. 1799–1809, 1995, doi: 10.1093/hmg/4.suppl_1.1799.

[70]   C. M. Kielty, "Elastic fibres in health and disease," *Expert Rev. Mol. Med.*, vol.

8, no. 19, pp. 1–23, 2006, doi: 10.1017/S146239940600007X.

[71]   L. Zacchigna *et al.*, "Emilin1 links TGF-beta maturation to blood pressure

homeostasis.," *Cell*, vol. 124, no. 5, pp. 929–942, Mar. 2006, doi:

10.1016/j.cell.2005.12.035.

[72] S. M. Arribas, A. Hinek, and M. C. González, "Elastic fibres and vascular structure in hypertension.," *Pharmacol. Ther.*, vol. 111, no. 3, pp. 771–791, Sep. 2006, doi: 10.1016/j.pharmthera.2005.12.003.

[73] T. Akima, K. Nakanishi, K. Suzuki, M. Katayama, F. Ohsuzu, and T. Kawai, "Soluble elastin decreases in the progress of atheroma formation in human aorta.," *Circ. J.*, vol. 73, no. 11, pp. 2154–2162, Nov. 2009, doi: 10.1253/circj.cj-09-0104.

[74] A. C. Newby, "Metalloproteinase production from macrophages - a perfect storm leading to atherosclerotic plaque rupture and myocardial infarction.," *Exp. Physiol.*, vol. 101, no. 11, pp. 1327–1337, Nov. 2016, doi: 10.1113/EP085567.

[75] J.-C. Lafarge, N. Naour, K. Clément, and M. Guerre-Millo, "Cathepsins and cystatin C in atherosclerosis and obesity.," *Biochimie*, vol. 92, no. 11, pp. 1580–1586, Nov. 2010, doi: 10.1016/j.biochi.2010.04.011.

[76] C. Van der Donckt *et al.*, "Elastin fragmentation in atherosclerotic mice leads to intraplaque neovascularization, plaque rupture, myocardial infarction, stroke, and sudden death," *Eur. Heart J.*, vol. 36, no. 17, pp. 1049–1058, Feb. 2014, doi: 10.1093/eurheartj/ehu041.

[77] J. S. Campa, R. M. Greenhalgh, and J. T. Powell, "Elastin degradation in abdominal aortic aneurysms.," *Atherosclerosis*, vol. 65, no. 1–2, pp. 13–21, May 1987, doi: 10.1016/0021-9150(87)90003-7.

[78] D. M. Milewicz *et al.*, "Genetic basis of thoracic aortic aneurysms and dissections: focus on smooth muscle cell contractile dysfunction.," *Annu. Rev.*

Genomics Hum. Genet., vol. 9, pp. 283–302, 2008, doi: 10.1146/annurev.genom.8.080706.092303.

[79]   V. Hucthagowder, N. Sausgruber, K. H. Kim, B. Angle, L. Y. Marmorstein, and Z. Urban, "Fibulin-4 : A Novel Gene for an Autosomal Recessive Cutis Laxa Syndrome," vol. 78, no. June, pp. 1075–1080, 2006.

[80]   G. Dong-chuan *et al.*, "LOX Mutations Predispose to Thoracic Aortic Aneurysms and Dissections," *Circ. Res.*, vol. 118, no. 6, pp. 928–934, Mar. 2016, doi: 10.1161/CIRCRESAHA.115.307130.

[81]   "Aorta Anatomy." [Online]. Available: https://ufhealth.org/uf-health-aortic-disease-center/aorta-anatomy.

[82]   A. Patel, B. Fine, M. Sandig, and K. Mequanint, "Elastin biosynthesis: The missing link in tissue-engineered blood vessels," *Cardiovasc. Res.*, vol. 71, no. 1, pp. 40–49, 2006, doi: 10.1016/j.cardiores.2006.02.021.

[83]   R. Ross, "The pathogenesis of atherosclerosis: a perspective for the 1990s.," *Nature*, vol. 362, no. 6423, pp. 801–809, Apr. 1993, doi: 10.1038/362801a0.

[84]   K. S. Bohl and J. L. West, "Nitric oxide-generating polymers reduce platelet adhesion and smooth muscle cell proliferation.," *Biomaterials*, vol. 21, no. 22, pp. 2273–2278, Nov. 2000, doi: 10.1016/s0142-9612(00)00153-8.

[85]   L. Junqueira and J. Carneiro, "Basic Histology: text and atlas," in *11th Edition*, 2008, pp. 206–207.

[86]   A. J. Cocciolone, J. Z. Hawes, M. C. Staiculescu, E. O. Johnson, M. Murshed, and J. E. Wagenseil, "Elastin , arterial mechanics , and cardiovascular disease,"

Am J Physiol Hear. Circ Physiol, vol. 315, pp. H189–H205, 2018, doi: 10.1152/ajpheart.00087.2018.

[87]   J. D'Armiento, "Decreased elastin in vessel walls puts the pressure on.," *J. Clin. Invest.*, vol. 112, no. 9, pp. 1308–1310, Nov. 2003, doi: 10.1172/JCI20226.

[88]   G. K. Owens, M. S. Kumar, and B. R. Wamhoff, "Molecular regulation of vascular smooth muscle cell differentiation in development and disease.," *Physiol. Rev.*, vol. 84, no. 3, pp. 767–801, Jul. 2004, doi: 10.1152/physrev.00041.2003.

[89]   G. K. Owens, "Role of mechanical strain in regulation of differentiation of vascular smooth muscle cells.," *Circulation research*, vol. 79, no. 5. United States, pp. 1054–1055, Nov-1996, doi: 10.1161/01.res.79.5.1054.

[90]   J. P. Stegemann, H. Hong, and R. M. Nerem, "Mechanical, biochemical, and extracellular matrix effects on vascular smooth muscle cell phenotype.," *J. Appl. Physiol.*, vol. 98, no. 6, pp. 2321–2327, Jun. 2005, doi: 10.1152/japplphysiol.01114.2004.

[91]   L. Robert, "Cell-elastin interaction and signaling.," *Pathol. Biol. (Paris).*, vol. 53, no. 7, pp. 399–404, Sep. 2005, doi: 10.1016/j.patbio.2004.12.020.

[92]   S. K. Karnik *et al.*, "A critical role for elastin signaling in vascular morphogenesis and disease.," *Development*, vol. 130, no. 2, pp. 411–423, Jan. 2003, doi: 10.1242/dev.00223.

[93]   A. Sourabh *et al.*, "Abdominal aortic aneurysm : A comprehensive review,"

Exp Clin Cardiol, vol. 16, no. 1, pp. 11–15, 2011.

[94]   X. Li, G. Zhao, J. Zhang, Z. Duan, and S. Xin, "Prevalence and Trends of the Abdominal Aortic Aneurysms Epidemic in General Population - A Meta-Analysis," *PLoS One*, vol. 8, no. 12, pp. 1–11, 2013, doi: 10.1371/journal.pone.0081260.

[95]   F. Lederle, G. Johnson, S. Wilson, E. Chute, F. Littooy, and B. D, "Prevalence and associations of abdominal aortic aneurysm detected through screening. Aneurysm Detection and Management," *Ann Intern Med*, vol. 126, no. 6, pp. 441–449, 1997.

[96]   A. B. Wilmink and C. R. Quick, "Epidemiology and potential for prevention of abdominal aortic aneurysm.," *Br. J. Surg.*, vol. 85, no. 2, pp. 155–162, Feb. 1998, doi: 10.1046/j.1365-2168.1998.00714.x.

[97]   L. J. 3rd Melton *et al.*, "Changing incidence of abdominal aortic aneurysms: a population-based study.," *Am. J. Epidemiol.*, vol. 120, no. 3, pp. 379–386, Sep. 1984, doi: 10.1093/oxfordjournals.aje.a113902.

[98]   W. M. Castleden and J. C. Mercer, "Abdominal aortic aneurysms in Western Australia: descriptive epidemiology and patterns of rupture.," *Br. J. Surg.*, vol. 72, no. 2, pp. 109–112, Feb. 1985, doi: 10.1002/bjs.1800720213.

[99]   R. F. Gillum, "Epidemiology of aortic aneurysm in the United States.," *J. Clin. Epidemiol.*, vol. 48, no. 11, pp. 1289–1298, Nov. 1995, doi: 10.1016/0895-4356(95)00045-3.

[100] C. Fleming, E. P. Whitlock, T. L. Beil, and F. A. Lederle, "Screening for

abdominal aortic aneurysm: a best-evidence systematic review for the U.S. Preventive Services Task Force.," *Ann. Intern. Med.*, vol. 142, no. 3, pp. 203–211, Feb. 2005, doi: 10.7326/0003-4819-142-3-200502010-00012.

[101] J. H. Lindeman and J. S. Matsumura, "Pharmacologic Management of Aneurysms," *Circ. Res.*, vol. 124, pp. 631–646, 2019, doi: 10.1161/CIRCRESAHA.118.312439.

[102] H. Aoki, Y. Ikeda, A. Furutani, and K. Hamano, "Development of pharmacological therapy for abdominal aortic aneurysms based on animal studies," in *Aortic Aneurysms, New Insights into An Old Problem*, 2008, pp. 453–476.

[103] H. Aoki, K. Yoshimura, and M. Matsuzaki, "Turning back the clock: regression of abdominal aortic aneurysms via pharmacotherapy.," *J. Mol. Med. (Berl).*, vol. 85, no. 10, pp. 1077–1088, Oct. 2007, doi: 10.1007/s00109-007-0213-2.

[104] R. W. Thompson, P. J. Geraghty, and J. K. Lee, "Abdominal aortic aneurysms: basic mechanisms and clinical implications.," *Curr. Probl. Surg.*, vol. 39, no. 2, pp. 110–230, Feb. 2002, doi: 10.1067/msg.2002.121421.

[105] S. Anidjar, P. B. Dobrin, M. Eichorst, G. P. Graham, and G. Chejfec, "Correlation of inflammatory infiltrate with the enlargement of experimental aortic aneurysms.," *J. Vasc. Surg.*, vol. 16, no. 2, pp. 139–147, Aug. 1992, doi: 10.1067/mva.1992.35585.

[106] E. L. Henderson, Y. J. Geng, G. K. Sukhova, A. D. Whittemore, J. Knox, and P. Libby, "Death of smooth muscle cells and expression of mediators of

apoptosis by T lymphocytes in human abdominal aortic aneurysms.,"
Circulation, vol. 99, no. 1, pp. 96–104, Jan. 1999, doi: 10.1161/01.cir.99.1.96.

[107] R. W. Thompson, S. Liao, and J. A. Curci, "Vascular smooth muscle cell apoptosis in abdominal aortic aneurysms.," *Coron. Artery Dis.*, vol. 8, no. 10, pp. 623–631, Oct. 1997, doi: 10.1097/00019501-199710000-00005.

[108] K. Shimizu, R. N. Mitchell, and P. Libby, "Inflammation and cellular immune responses in abdominal aortic aneurysms.," *Arterioscler. Thromb. Vasc. Biol.*, vol. 26, no. 5, pp. 987–994, May 2006, doi: 10.1161/01.ATV.0000214999.12921.4f.

[109] J. Sun *et al.*, "Mast cells modulate the pathogenesis of elastase-induced abdominal aortic aneurysms in mice.," *J. Clin. Invest.*, vol. 117, no. 11, pp. 3359–3368, Nov. 2007, doi: 10.1172/JCI31311.

[110] K. Yoshimura and H. Aoki, "Recent Advances in Pharmacotherapy Development for Abdominal Aortic Aneurysm," *Int. J. Vasc. Med.*, vol. 2012, no. 648167, pp. 1–9, 2012, doi: 10.1155/2012/648167.

[111] A. Daugherty and L. A. Cassis, "Mechanisms of abdominal aortic aneurysm formation.," *Curr. Atheroscler. Rep.*, vol. 4, no. 3, pp. 222–227, May 2002, doi: 10.1007/s11883-002-0023-5.

[112] I. M. Nordon, R. J. Hinchliffe, I. M. Loftus, and M. M. Thompson, "Pathophysiology and epidemiology of abdominal aortic aneurysms.," *Nat. Rev. Cardiol.*, vol. 8, no. 2, pp. 92–102, Feb. 2011, doi: 10.1038/nrcardio.2010.180.

[113] M. D. Huffman, J. A. Curci, G. Moore, D. B. Kerns, B. C. Starcher, and R. W. Thompson, "Functional importance of connective tissue repair during the development of experimental abdominal aortic aneurysms.," *Surgery*, vol. 128, no. 3, pp. 429–38, 2000, doi: 10.1067/msy.2000.107379.

[114] M. Rentschler and B. T. Baxter, "Pharmacological approaches to prevent abdominal aortic aneurysm enlargement and rupture.," *Ann. N. Y. Acad. Sci.*, vol. 1085, pp. 39–46, Nov. 2006, doi: 10.1196/annals.1383.003.

[115] A. R. Brady, S. G. Thompson, F. G. R. Fowkes, R. M. Greenhalgh, and J. T. Powell, "Abdominal aortic aneurysm expansion: risk factors and time intervals for surveillance.," *Circulation*, vol. 110, no. 1, pp. 16–21, Jul. 2004, doi: 10.1161/01.CIR.0000133279.07468.9F.

[116] T. Fülöp *et al.*, "[The elastin-laminin receptor].," *J. Soc. Biol.*, vol. 195, no. 2, pp. 157–164, 2001.

[117] F. A. M. V. I. Hellenthal, I. L. A. Geenen, J. A. W. Teijink, S. Heeneman, and G. W. H. Schurink, "Histological features of human abdominal aortic aneurysm are not related to clinical characteristics.," *Cardiovasc. Pathol. Off. J. Soc. Cardiovasc. Pathol.*, vol. 18, no. 5, pp. 286–293, 2009, doi: 10.1016/j.carpath.2008.06.014.

[118] G. T. Jones, "The Pathohistology of Abdominal Aortic Aneurysm," in *Diagnosis, Screening and Treatment of Abdominal, Thoracoabdominal and Thoracic Aortic Aneurysms*, 2011, pp. 53–73.

[119] F. A. M. V. I. Hellenthal, I. L. A. Geenen, J. A. W. Teijink, G. W. H. Schurink, and S. Heeneman, "Histological features of human abdominal aortic aneurysm

are not related to clinical characteristics," *Cardiovasc. Pathol.*, vol. 18, no. 5, pp. 286–293, 2009, doi: 10.1016/j.carpath.2008.06.014.

[120] D. C. Brewster, J. L. Cronenwett, J. W. Hallett, K. W. Johnston, W. C. Krupski, and J. S. Matsumura, "Guidelines for the treatment of abdominal aortic aneurysms: Report of a subcommittee of the Joint Council of the American Association for Vascular Surgery and Society for Vascular Surgery," *J. Vasc. Surg.*, vol. 37, no. 5, pp. 1106–17, 2003, doi: 10.1067/mva.2003.363.

[121] D. E. Szilagyi, R. F. Smith, F. J. DeRusso, J. P. Elliott, and F. W. Sherrin, "Contribution of abdominal aortic aneurysmectomy to prolongation of life.," *Ann. Surg.*, vol. 164, no. 4, pp. 678–699, Oct. 1966, doi: 10.1097/00000658-196610000-00014.

[122] N. J. Swerdlow, W. W. Wu, and M. L. Schermerhorn, "Open and Endovascular Management of Aortic Aneurysms," *Circ. Res.*, vol. 124, pp. 647–661, 2019, doi: 10.1161/CIRCRESAHA.118.313186.

[123] A. Karthikesalingam *et al.*, "Mortality from ruptured abdominal aortic aneurysms: clinical lessons from a comparison of outcomes in England and the USA.," *Lancet (London, England)*, vol. 383, no. 9921, pp. 963–969, Mar. 2014, doi: 10.1016/S0140-6736(14)60109-4.

[124] B. Amato *et al.*, "Endovascular repair versus open repair in the treatment of ruptured aortic aneurysms : a systematic review," *Minerva Chir.*, vol. 74, no. 6, pp. 472–480, 2019, doi: 10.23736/S0026-4733.18.07768-4.

[125] M. E. Törnwall, J. Virtamo, J. K. Haukka, D. Albanes, and J. K. Huttunen, "Alpha-tocopherol (vitamin E) and beta-carotene supplementation does not

affect the risk for large abdominal aortic aneurysm in a controlled trial.,"
Atherosclerosis, vol. 157, no. 1, pp. 167–173, Jul. 2001, doi: 10.1016/s0021-
9150(00)00694-8.

[126] D. Gavrila *et al.*, "Vitamin E inhibits abdominal aortic aneurysm formation in
angiotensin II-infused apolipoprotein E-deficient mice.," *Arterioscler.
Thromb. Vasc. Biol.*, vol. 25, no. 8, pp. 1671–1677, Aug. 2005, doi:
10.1161/01.ATV.0000172631.50972.0f.

[127] S. Liao, M. Miralles, B. J. Kelley, J. A. Curci, M. Borhani, and R. W.
Thompson, "Suppression of experimental abdominal aortic aneurysms in the
rat by treatment with angiotensin-converting enzyme inhibitors.," *J. Vasc.
Surg.*, vol. 33, no. 5, pp. 1057–1064, May 2001, doi:
10.1067/mva.2001.112810.

[128] A. Kalyanasundaram *et al.*, "Simvastatin suppresses experimental aortic
aneurysm expansion.," *J. Vasc. Surg.*, vol. 43, no. 1, pp. 117–124, Jan. 2006,
doi: 10.1016/j.jvs.2005.08.007.

[129] E. F. Steinmetz *et al.*, "Treatment with simvastatin suppresses the development
of experimental abdominal aortic aneurysms in normal and
hypercholesterolemic mice.," *Ann. Surg.*, vol. 241, no. 1, pp. 92–101, Jan.
2005, doi: 10.1097/01.sla.0000150258.36236.e0.

[130] Y. Wang *et al.*, "TGF-beta activity protects against inflammatory aortic
aneurysm progression and complications in angiotensin II-infused mice.," *J.
Clin. Invest.*, vol. 120, no. 2, pp. 422–432, Feb. 2010, doi: 10.1172/JCI38136.

[131] A. Hata and Y.-G. Chen, "TGF-β Signaling from Receptors to Smads.," *Cold*

Spring Harb. Perspect. Biol., vol. 8, no. 9, Sep. 2016, doi: 10.1101/cshperspect.a022061.

[132] C. P. Hans *et al.*, "Inhibition of Notch1 Signaling Reduces Abdominal Aortic Aneruysm in Mice by Attenuating Macrophage-Mediated Inflammation," *Arterioscler. Thromb. Vasc. Biol.*, vol. 32, no. 12, pp. 3012–3023, 2012, doi: 10.1161/ATVBAHA.112.254219.Inhibition.

[133] F. J. J. Miller, W. J. Sharp, X. Fang, L. W. Oberley, T. D. Oberley, and N. L. Weintraub, "Oxidative stress in human abdominal aortic aneurysms: a potential mediator of aneurysmal remodeling.," *Arterioscler. Thromb. Vasc. Biol.*, vol. 22, no. 4, pp. 560–565, Apr. 2002, doi: 10.1161/01.atv.0000013778.72404.30.

[134] A. H. Sprague and R. A. Khalil, "Inflammatory cytokines in vascular dysfunction and vascular disease.," *Biochem. Pharmacol.*, vol. 78, no. 6, pp. 539–552, Sep. 2009, doi: 10.1016/j.bcp.2009.04.029.

[135] W. Xiong *et al.*, "Inhibition of reactive oxygen species attenuates aneurysm formation in a murine model," *Atherosclerosis*, vol. 202, no. 1, pp. 128–134, 2009, doi: 10.1016/j.atherosclerosis.2008.03.029.Inhibition.

[136] X.-F. Lei *et al.*, "Identification of Hic-5 as a novel scaffold for the MKK4/p54 JNK pathway in the development of abdominal aortic aneurysms.," *J. Am. Heart Assoc.*, vol. 3, no. 3, p. e000747, May 2014, doi: 10.1161/JAHA.113.000747.

[137] F. M. Davis, D. L. Rateri, and A. Daugherty, "Abdominal Aortic Aneurysm: Novel Mechanism and Therapies," *Curr Opin Cardiol.*, vol. 30, no. 6, pp. 566–573, 2015, doi: 10.1097/HCO.0000000000000216.Abdominal.

[138] L. Maegdefessel *et al.*, "Inhibition of microRNA-29b reduces murine abdominal aortic aneurysm development," *J. Clin. Invest.*, vol. 122, no. 2, pp. 497–506, 2012, doi: 10.1172/JCI61598.

[139] L. Maegdefessel *et al.*, "MicroRNA-21 blocks abdominal aortic aneurysm development and nicotine-augmented expansion.," *Sci. Transl. Med.*, vol. 4, no. 122, p. 122ra22, Feb. 2012, doi: 10.1126/scitranslmed.3003441.

[140] L. Maegdefessel *et al.*, "miR-24 limits aortic vascular inflammation and murine abdominal aneurysm development.," *Nat. Commun.*, vol. 5, p. 5214, Oct. 2014, doi: 10.1038/ncomms6214.

[141] C. Luna, G. Li, J. Qiu, D. L. Epstein, and P. Gonzalez, "Cross-talk between miR-29 and transforming growth factor-betas in trabecular meshwork cells.," *Invest. Ophthalmol. Vis. Sci.*, vol. 52, no. 6, pp. 3567–3572, Jun. 2011, doi: 10.1167/iovs.10-6448.

[142] S. M. Hawkins *et al.*, "Functional microRNA involved in endometriosis.," *Mol. Endocrinol.*, vol. 25, no. 5, pp. 821–832, May 2011, doi: 10.1210/me.2010-0371.

[143] R. Steele, J. L. Mott, and R. B. Ray, "MBP-1 upregulates miR-29b that represses Mcl-1, collagens, and matrix-metalloproteinase-2 in prostate cancer cells.," *Genes Cancer*, vol. 1, no. 4, pp. 381–387, Apr. 2010, doi: 10.1177/1947601910371978.

[144] Z. Li *et al.*, "Biological functions of miR-29b contribute to positive regulation of osteoblast differentiation.," *J. Biol. Chem.*, vol. 284, no. 23, pp. 15676–15684, Jun. 2009, doi: 10.1074/jbc.M809787200.

[145] L. Maegdefessel, J. Azuma, and P. S. Tsao, "MicroRNA-29b regulation of abdominal aortic aneurysm development," *Trends Cardiovasc Med.*, vol. 24, no. 1, pp. 1–10, 2015, doi: 10.1016/j.tcm.2013.05.002.MicroRNA-29b.

[146] Y. Dorsett and T. Tuschl, "siRNAs: applications in functional genomics and potential as therapeutics.," *Nat. Rev. Drug Discov.*, vol. 3, no. 4, pp. 318–329, Apr. 2004, doi: 10.1038/nrd1345.

[147] S. M. Elbashir, J. Harborth, W. Lendeckel, A. Yalcin, K. Weber, and T. Tuschl, "Duplexes of 21-nucleotide RNAs mediate RNA interference in cultured mammalian cells.," *Nature*, vol. 411, no. 6836, pp. 494–498, May 2001, doi: 10.1038/35078107.

[148] P. D. Zamore, T. Tuschl, P. A. Sharp, and D. P. Bartel, "RNAi: double-stranded RNA directs the ATP-dependent cleavage of mRNA at 21 to 23 nucleotide intervals.," *Cell*, vol. 101, no. 1, pp. 25–33, Mar. 2000, doi: 10.1016/S0092-8674(00)80620-0.

[149] Y. Zhang, "RNA-induced Silencing Complex (RISC) BT - Encyclopedia of Systems Biology," W. Dubitzky, O. Wolkenhauer, K.-H. Cho, and H. Yokota, Eds. New York, NY: Springer New York, 2013, p. 1876.

[150] R. Majumdar, K. Rajasekaran, and J. W. Cary, "RNA Interference (RNAi) as a Potential Tool for Control of Mycotoxin Contamination in Crop Plants: Concepts and Considerations," *Front. Plant Sci.*, vol. 8, p. 200, 2017, doi: 10.3389/fpls.2017.00200.

[151] X. Su, L. Ao, Y. Shi, T. R. Johnson, D. A. Fullerton, and X. Meng, "Oxidized low density lipoprotein induces bone morphogenetic protein-2 in coronary

artery endothelial cells via Toll-like receptors 2 and 4.," *J. Biol. Chem.*, vol. 286, no. 14, pp. 12213–12220, Apr. 2011, doi: 10.1074/jbc.M110.214619.

[152] X. W. Cheng *et al.*, "Angiotensin type 1 receptor blocker reduces intimal neovascularization and plaque growth in apolipoprotein E-deficient mice.," *Hypertens. (Dallas, Tex. 1979)*, vol. 57, no. 5, pp. 981–989, May 2011, doi: 10.1161/HYPERTENSIONAHA.110.168385.

[153] V. de Waard *et al.*, "Systemic MCP1/CCR2 blockade and leukocyte specific MCP1/CCR2 inhibition affect aortic aneurysm formation differently.," *Atherosclerosis*, vol. 211, no. 1, pp. 84–89, Jul. 2010, doi: 10.1016/j.atherosclerosis.2010.01.042.

[154] J. Cao *et al.*, "Spatiotemporal expression of matrix metalloproteinases (MMPs) is regulated by the Ca2+-signal transducer S100A4 in the pathogenesis of thoracic aortic aneurysm.," *PLoS One*, vol. 8, no. 7, p. e70057, 2013, doi: 10.1371/journal.pone.0070057.

[155] Z. Liu *et al.*, "Hyperhomocysteinemia exaggerates adventitial inflammation and angiotensin II-induced abdominal aortic aneurysm in mice.," *Circ. Res.*, vol. 111, no. 10, pp. 1261–1273, Oct. 2012, doi: 10.1161/CIRCRESAHA.112.270520.

[156] M. Salmon *et al.*, "KLF4 regulates abdominal aortic aneurysm morphology and deletion attenuates aneurysm formation.," *Circulation*, vol. 128, no. 11 Suppl 1, pp. S163-74, Sep. 2013, doi: 10.1161/CIRCULATIONAHA.112.000238.

[157] A. Dwivedi, S. C. Slater, and S. J. George, "MMP-9 and -12 cause N-cadherin shedding and thereby beta-catenin signalling and vascular smooth muscle cell

proliferation.," *Cardiovasc. Res.*, vol. 81, no. 1, pp. 178–186, Jan. 2009, doi: 10.1093/cvr/cvn278.

[158] A. Ghosh *et al.*, "The role of extracellular signal-related kinase during abdominal aortic aneurysm formation.," *J. Am. Coll. Surg.*, vol. 215, no. 5, pp. 668-680.e1, Nov. 2012, doi: 10.1016/j.jamcollsurg.2012.06.414.

[159] P. D. DiMusto *et al.*, "Increased JNK in males compared with females in a rodent model of abdominal aortic aneurysm.," *J. Surg. Res.*, vol. 176, no. 2, pp. 687–695, Aug. 2012, doi: 10.1016/j.jss.2011.11.1024.

[160] F. Jung, J. Haendeler, C. Goebel, A. M. Zeiher, and S. Dimmeler, "Growth factor-induced phosphoinositide 3-OH kinase/Akt phosphorylation in smooth muscle cells: induction of cell proliferation and inhibition of cell death.," *Cardiovasc. Res.*, vol. 48, no. 1, pp. 148–157, Oct. 2000, doi: 10.1016/s0008-6363(00)00152-8.

[161] L. Pradhan-Nabzdyk, C. Huang, F. W. Logerfo, and C. S. Nabzdyk, "Current siRNA Targets in Atherosclerosis and Aortic Aneurysm," *Discov Med.*, vol. 17, no. 95, pp. 233–246, 2014.

[162] M. A. DePristo *et al.*, "A framework for variation discovery and genotyping using next-generation DNA sequencing data.," *Nat. Genet.*, vol. 43, no. 5, pp. 491–498, May 2011, doi: 10.1038/ng.806.

[163] A. Camardo, D. Seshadri, T. Broekelmann, R. Mecham, and A. Ramamurthi, "Multifunctional, JNK-inhibiting nanotherapeutics for augmented elastic matrix regenerative repair in aortic aneurysms," *Drug Deliv. Transl. Res.*, vol. 8, no. 4, pp. 964–984, 2018, doi: 10.1007/s13346-017-0419-y.

[164] B. Jennewine, J. Fox, and A. Ramamurthi, "Cathepsin K-targeted sub-micron particles for regenerative repair of vascular elastic matrix," *Acta Biomater.*, vol. 52, pp. 60–73, 2017, doi: 10.1016/j.actbio.2017.01.032.

[165] J. A. Beamish, P. He, K. Kottke-Marchant, and R. E. Marchant, "Molecular Regulation of Contractile Smooth Muscle Cell Phenotype: Implications for Vascular Tissue Engineering," *Tissue Eng. Part B Rev.*, vol. 16, no. 5, pp. 467–491, Mar. 2010, doi: 10.1089/ten.teb.2009.0630.

[166] C. E. Gacchina, P. Deb, J. L. Barth, and A. Ramamurthi, "Elastogenic inductability of smooth muscle cells from a rat model of late stage abdominal aortic aneurysms.," *Tissue Eng. Part A*, vol. 17, no. 13–14, pp. 1699–711, 2011, doi: 10.1089/ten.TEA.2010.0526.

[167] C. Gacchina, T. Brothers, and A. Ramamurthi, "Evaluating smooth muscle cells from CaCl2-induced rat aortal expansions as a surrogate culture model for study of elastogenic induction of human aneurysmal cells.," *Tissue Eng. Part A*, vol. 17, no. 15–16, pp. 1945–58, 2011, doi: 10.1089/ten.TEA.2010.0475.

[168] C. R. Kothapalli, P. M. Taylor, R. T. Smolenski, M. H. Yacoub, and A. Ramamurthi, "Transforming Growth Factor Beta 1 and Hyaluronan Oligomers Synergistically Enhance Elastin Matrix Regeneration by Vascular Smooth Muscle Cells," *Tissue Eng. Part A*, vol. 15, no. 3, pp. 501–511, Oct. 2008, doi: 10.1089/ten.tea.2008.0040.

[169] R. A. Boon and S. Dimmeler, "MicroRNAs and Aneurysm Formation," *Trends Cardiovasc. Med.*, vol. 21, no. 6, pp. 172–177, 2011, doi: https://doi.org/10.1016/j.tcm.2012.05.005.

[170] E. Allaire *et al.*, "Vascular smooth muscle cell endovascular therapy stabilizes already developed aneurysms in a model of aortic injury elicited by inflammation and proteolysis," *Ann. Surg.*, vol. 239, no. 3, pp. 417–427, Mar. 2004, doi: 10.1097/01.sla.0000114131.79899.82.

[171] G. Kolios and Y. Moodley, "Introduction to stem cells and regenerative medicine," *Respiration*, vol. 85, no. 1, pp. 3–10, 2012, doi: 10.1159/000345615.

[172] A. Smith, "A Glossary for Stem Cell Biology," *Nature*, vol. 441, no. 29, p. 1060, 2006.

[173] J. Rossant, "Stem cells from the Mammalian blastocyst.," *Stem Cells*, vol. 19, no. 6, pp. 477–482, 2001, doi: 10.1634/stemcells.19-6-477.

[174] M. P. De Miguel, S. Fuentes-Julián, and Y. Alcaina, "Pluripotent stem cells: origin, maintenance and induction.," *Stem cell Rev. reports*, vol. 6, no. 4, pp. 633–649, Dec. 2010, doi: 10.1007/s12015-010-9170-1.

[175] A. Augello, T. B. Kurth, and C. De Bari, "Mesenchymal stem cells: a perspective from in vitro cultures to in vivo migration and niches.," *Eur. Cell. Mater.*, vol. 20, pp. 121–133, Sep. 2010, doi: 10.22203/ecm.v020a11.

[176] M. Z. Ratajczak, E. Zuba-Surma, M. Kucia, A. Poniewierska, M. Suszynska, and J. Ratajczak, "Pluripotent and multipotent stem cells in adult tissues.," *Adv. Med. Sci.*, vol. 57, no. 1, pp. 1–17, Jun. 2012, doi: 10.2478/v10039-012-0020-z.

[177] F. Majo, A. Rochat, M. Nicolas, G. A. Jaoudé, and Y. Barrandon, "Oligopotent

stem cells are distributed throughout the mammalian ocular surface.," *Nature*, vol. 456, no. 7219, pp. 250–254, Nov. 2008, doi: 10.1038/nature07406.

[178] M. Marone *et al.*, "Cell cycle regulation in human hematopoietic stem cells: from isolation to activation.," *Leuk. Lymphoma*, vol. 43, no. 3, pp. 493–501, Mar. 2002, doi: 10.1080/10428190290011967.

[179] K. Overturf, M. al-Dhalimy, C. N. Ou, M. Finegold, and M. Grompe, "Serial transplantation reveals the stem-cell-like regenerative potential of adult mouse hepatocytes.," *Am. J. Pathol.*, vol. 151, no. 5, pp. 1273–1280, Nov. 1997.

[180] D. G. de Rooij and J. A. Grootegoed, "Spermatogonial stem cells.," *Curr. Opin. Cell Biol.*, vol. 10, no. 6, pp. 694–701, Dec. 1998, doi: 10.1016/s0955-0674(98)80109-9.

[181] C. F. Bentzinger, Y. X. Wang, J. von Maltzahn, and M. A. Rudnicki, "The emerging biology of muscle stem cells: implications for cell-based therapies.," *Bioessays*, vol. 35, no. 3, pp. 231–241, Mar. 2013, doi: 10.1002/bies.201200063.

[182] B. Beck and C. Blanpain, "Mechanisms regulating epidermal stem cells.," *EMBO J.*, vol. 31, no. 9, pp. 2067–2075, May 2012, doi: 10.1038/emboj.2012.67.

[183] S. Yao *et al.*, "Long-term self-renewal and directed differentiation of human embryonic stem cells in chemically defined conditions.," *Proc. Natl. Acad. Sci. U. S. A.*, vol. 103, no. 18, pp. 6907–6912, May 2006, doi: 10.1073/pnas.0602280103.

[184] M. J. Evans and M. H. Kaufman, "Establishment in culture of pluripotential cells from mouse embryos," *Nature*, vol. 292, no. 5819, pp. 154–156, 1981, doi: 10.1038/292154a0.

[185] Z. Wang, E. Oron, B. Nelson, S. Razis, and N. Ivanova, "Distinct lineage specification roles for NANOG, OCT4, and SOX2 in human embryonic stem cells.," *Cell Stem Cell*, vol. 10, no. 4, pp. 440–454, Apr. 2012, doi: 10.1016/j.stem.2012.02.016.

[186] F. Hambiliki, S. Ström, P. Zhang, and A. Stavreus-Evers, "Co-localization of NANOG and OCT4 in human pre-implantation embryos and in human embryonic stem cells.," *J. Assist. Reprod. Genet.*, vol. 29, no. 10, pp. 1021–1028, Oct. 2012, doi: 10.1007/s10815-012-9824-9.

[187] S. Ilancheran, Y. Moodley, and U. Manuelpillai, "Human fetal membranes: a source of stem cells for tissue regeneration and repair?," *Placenta*, vol. 30, no. 1, pp. 2–10, Jan. 2009, doi: 10.1016/j.placenta.2008.09.009.

[188] M. Körbling and Z. Estrov, "Adult stem cells for tissue repair - a new therapeutic concept?," *N. Engl. J. Med.*, vol. 349, no. 6, pp. 570–582, Aug. 2003, doi: 10.1056/NEJMra022361.

[189] J. B. McCormick and H. A. Huso, "Stem cells and ethics: current issues.," *J. Cardiovasc. Transl. Res.*, vol. 3, no. 2, pp. 122–127, Apr. 2010, doi: 10.1007/s12265-009-9155-0.

[190] R. Passier and C. Mummery, "Origin and use of embryonic and adult stem cells in differentiation and tissue repair.," *Cardiovasc. Res.*, vol. 58, no. 2, pp. 324–335, May 2003, doi: 10.1016/s0008-6363(02)00770-8.

[191] J. Voog and D. L. Jones, "Stem cells and the niche: a dynamic duo.," *Cell Stem Cell*, vol. 6, no. 2, pp. 103–115, Feb. 2010, doi: 10.1016/j.stem.2010.01.011.

[192] N. Smart and P. R. Riley, "The stem cell movement.," *Circ. Res.*, vol. 102, no. 10, pp. 1155–1168, May 2008, doi: 10.1161/CIRCRESAHA.108.175158.

[193] T. M. Yeung, L. A. Chia, C. M. Kosinski, and C. J. Kuo, "Regulation of self-renewal and differentiation by the intestinal stem cell niche.," *Cell. Mol. Life Sci.*, vol. 68, no. 15, pp. 2513–2523, Aug. 2011, doi: 10.1007/s00018-011-0687-5.

[194] J. C. Kiefer, "Primer and interviews: The dynamic stem cell niche.," *Dev. Dyn. an Off. Publ. Am. Assoc. Anat.*, vol. 240, no. 3, pp. 737–743, Mar. 2011, doi: 10.1002/dvdy.22566.

[195] J. Rossant, "Stem cells and early lineage development.," *Cell*, vol. 132, no. 4, pp. 527–531, Feb. 2008, doi: 10.1016/j.cell.2008.01.039.

[196] K. Takahashi *et al.*, "Induction of pluripotent stem cells from adult human fibroblasts by defined factors.," *Cell*, vol. 131, no. 5, pp. 861–872, Nov. 2007, doi: 10.1016/j.cell.2007.11.019.

[197] M. Stadtfeld, M. Nagaya, J. Utikal, G. Weir, and K. Hochedlinger, "Induced pluripotent stem cells generated without viral integration.," *Science*, vol. 322, no. 5903, pp. 945–949, Nov. 2008, doi: 10.1126/science.1162494.

[198] K. Okita, M. Nakagawa, H. Hyenjong, T. Ichisaka, and S. Yamanaka, "Generation of mouse induced pluripotent stem cells without viral vectors," *Science*, vol. 322, no. 5903, pp. 949–953, Nov. 2008, doi:

10.1126/science.1164270.

[199] K. Woltjen *et al.*, "piggyBac transposition reprograms fibroblasts to induced pluripotent stem cells.," *Nature*, vol. 458, no. 7239, pp. 766–770, Apr. 2009, doi: 10.1038/nature07863.

[200] K. Kaji, K. Norrby, A. Paca, M. Mileikovsky, P. Mohseni, and K. Woltjen, "Virus-free induction of pluripotency and subsequent excision of reprogramming factors.," *Nature*, vol. 458, no. 7239, pp. 771–775, Apr. 2009, doi: 10.1038/nature07864.

[201] A. J. Friedenstein, K. V Petrakova, A. I. Kurolesova, and G. P. Frolova, "Heterotopic of bone marrow. Analysis of precursor cells for osteogenic and hematopoietic tissues.," *Transplantation*, vol. 6, no. 2, pp. 230–247, Mar. 1968.

[202] U. Lindner, J. Kramer, J. Rohwedel, and P. Schlenke, "Mesenchymal stem or stromal cells: Toward a better understanding of their biology?," *Transfus. Med. Hemotherapy*, vol. 37, no. 2, pp. 75–83, 2010, doi: 10.1159/000290897.

[203] M. Krampera, J. Galipeau, Y. Shi, K. Tarte, and L. Sensebe, "Immunological characterization of multipotent mesenchymal stromal cells--The International Society for Cellular Therapy (ISCT) working proposal.," *Cytotherapy*, vol. 15, no. 9, pp. 1054–1061, Sep. 2013, doi: 10.1016/j.jcyt.2013.02.010.

[204] P. J. Simmons and B. Torok-Storb, "Identification of stromal cell precursors in human bone marrow by a novel monoclonal antibody, STRO-1.," *Blood*, vol. 78, no. 1, pp. 55–62, Jul. 1991.

[205] B. Sacchetti *et al.*, "Self-renewing osteoprogenitors in bone marrow sinusoids

can organize a hematopoietic microenvironment.," *Cell*, vol. 131, no. 2, pp. 324–336, Oct. 2007, doi: 10.1016/j.cell.2007.08.025.

[206] S. Gronthos *et al.*, "Molecular and cellular characterisation of highly purified stromal stem cells derived from human bone marrow.," *J. Cell Sci.*, vol. 116, no. Pt 9, pp. 1827–1835, May 2003, doi: 10.1242/jcs.00369.

[207] A. Andrzejewska, B. Lukomska, and M. Janowski, "Concise Review: Mesenchymal Stem Cells: From Roots to Boost," *Stem Cells*, vol. 37, no. 7, pp. 855–864, 2019, doi: 10.1002/stem.3016.

[208] D. Mushahary, A. Spittler, C. Kasper, V. Weber, and V. Charwat, "Isolation, cultivation, and characterization of human mesenchymal stem cells," *Cytom. Part A*, vol. 93, no. 1, pp. 19–31, 2018, doi: 10.1002/cyto.a.23242.

[209] P. P. Deb and A. Ramamurthi, "Spatiotemporal mapping of matrix remodelling and evidence of in situ elastogenesis in experimental abdominal aortic aneurysms," *J. Tissue Eng. Regen. Med.*, vol. 11, no. 1, pp. 231–245, 2017, doi: 10.1002/term.1905.

[210] C. A. Bashur and R. R. Rao, "Perspectives on Stem Cell-Based Elastic Matrix Regenerative Therapies for Abdominal Aortic Aneurysms," *Stem cells Transitional Med.*, vol. 2, pp. 401–408, 2013.

[211] M. Nakagawa *et al.*, "Generation of induced pluripotent stem cells without Myc from mouse and human fibroblasts.," *Nat. Biotechnol.*, vol. 26, no. 1, pp. 101–106, Jan. 2008, doi: 10.1038/nbt1374.

[212] A. Yamawaki-Ogata, R. Hashizume, X.-M. Fu, A. Usui, and Y. Narita,

"Mesenchymal stem cells for treatment of aortic aneurysms.," *World J. Stem Cells*, vol. 6, no. 3, pp. 278–87, 2014, doi: 10.4252/wjsc.v6.i3.278.

[213] J. Rossignol *et al.*, "Mesenchymal stem cells induce a weak immune response in the rat striatum after allo or xenotransplantation," *J. Cell. Mol. Med.*, vol. 13, no. 8 B, pp. 2547–2558, 2009, doi: 10.1111/j.1582-4934.2009.00657.x.

[214] G. Swaminathan, V. S. Gadepalli, I. Stoilov, R. P. Mecham, R. R. Rao, and A. Ramamurthi, "Pro-elastogenic effects of bone marrow mesenchymal stem cell-derived smooth muscle cells on cultured aneurysmal smooth muscle cells.," *J. Tissue Eng. Regen. Med.*, vol. 4, no. 7, pp. 524–31, 2014, doi: 10.1002/term.1964.

[215] G. Swaminathan, I. Stoilov, T. Broekelmann, R. Mecham, and A. Ramamurthi, "Phenotype-Based Selection of Bone Marrow Mesenchymal Stem Cell-Derived Smooth Muscle Cells for Elastic Matrix Regenerative Repair in Abdominal Aortic Aneurysms," *J. Tissue Eng. Regen. Med.*, 2016, doi: 10.1002/term.2349.

[216] X. Wei, X. Yang, Z. Han, F. Qu, L. Shao, and Y. Shi, "Mesenchymal stem cells: a new trend for cell therapy.," *Acta Pharmacol. Sin.*, vol. 34, no. 6, pp. 747–754, Jun. 2013, doi: 10.1038/aps.2013.50.

[217] A. Sohni and C. M. Verfaillie, "Mesenchymal stem cells migration homing and tracking," *Stem Cells Int.*, 2013, doi: 10.1155/2013/130763.

[218] R. F. Wynn *et al.*, "A small proportion of mesenchymal stem cells strongly expresses functionally active CXCR4 receptor capable of promoting migration to bone marrow," *Blood*, vol. 104, no. 9, pp. 2643–2645, 2004, doi:

10.1182/blood-2004-02-0526.

[219] S. Aggarwal, A. Qamar, V. Sharma, and A. Sharma, "Abdominal aortic aneurysm: A comprehensive review," *Experimental and Clinical Cardiology*. 2011.

[220] J. L. Eliason and G. R. Upchurch, "Endovascular Abdominal Aortic Aneurysm Repair," *Circulation*, vol. 117, no. 13, pp. 1738–1744, 2008, doi: 10.1161/CIRCULATIONAHA.107.747923.

[221] A. England and R. Mc Williams, "Endovascular aortic aneurysm repair (EVAR).," *Ulster Med. J.*, vol. 82, no. 1, pp. 3–10, 2013.

[222] C. A. Bashur, R. R. Rao, and A. Ramamurthi, "Perspectives on Stem Cell-Based Elastic Matrix Regenerative Therapies for Abdominal Aortic Aneurysms," *Stem Cells Transl. Med.*, vol. 2, no. 6, pp. 401–408, 2013, doi: 10.5966/sctm.2012-0185.

[223] G. K. Owens, "Regulation of differentiation of vascular smooth muscle cells," *Physiol. Rev.*, vol. 75, no. 3, pp. 487–517, 2017, doi: 10.1152/physrev.1995.75.3.487.

[224] J. P. Stegemann, H. Hong, R. M. Nerem, and P. Jan, "Mechanical, biochemical, and extracellular matrix effects on vascular smooth muscle cell phenotype," *J App Physiol*, vol. 98, no. 6, pp. 2321–2327, 2005, doi: 10.1152/japplphysiol.01114.2004.

[225] S. S. M. Rensen, P. A. F. M. Doevendans, and G. J. J. M. van Eys, "Regulation and characteristics of vascular smooth muscle cell phenotypic diversity.," *Neth.*

Heart J., vol. 15, no. 3, pp. 100–8, 2007, doi: 10.1007/BF03085963.

[226] C. R. Kothapalli and A. Ramamurthi, "Induced elastin regeneration by chronically activated smooth muscle cells for targeted aneurysm repair," *Acta Biomater.*, vol. 6, no. 1, pp. 170–178, 2010, doi: 10.1016/j.actbio.2009.06.006.

[227] M. W. Pfaffl, "A new mathematical model for relative quantification in real-time RT-PCR," *Nucleic Acids Res.*, vol. 29, no. 9, pp. 45e – 45, 2001, doi: 10.1093/nar/29.9.e45.

[228] B. Sivaraman *et al.*, "Magnetically-responsive, multifunctional drug delivery nanoparticles for elastic matrix regenerative repair," *Acta Biomater.*, vol. 52, 2017, doi: 10.1016/j.actbio.2016.11.048.

[229] C. Labarca and K. Paigen, "A simple, rapid, and sensitive DNA assay procedure," *Anal. Biochem.*, 1980, doi: 10.1016/0003-2697(80)90165-7.

[230] B. Starcher, "A ninhydrin-based assay to quantitate the total protein content of tissue samples.," *Anal. Biochem.*, vol. 292, no. 1, pp. 125–9, 2001, doi: 10.1006/abio.2001.5050.

[231] L. Venkataraman and A. Ramamurthi, "Induced Elastic Matrix Deposition Within Three-Dimensional Collagen Scaffolds," *Tissue Eng. Part A*, vol. 17, no. 21–22, pp. 2879–2889, 2011, doi: 10.1089/ten.tea.2010.0749.

[232] Novus Biologicals a biotechne brand, "Beta Actin and GAPDH: The Importance of Loading Controls | Antibody News: Novus Biologicals," *11/09/2011*, 2011. .

[233] Z. An *et al.*, "Interleukin-6 downregulated vascular smooth muscle cell

contractile proteins via ATG4B-mediated autophagy in thoracic aortic dissection," *Heart Vessels*, vol. 32, no. 12, pp. 1523–1535, 2017, doi: 10.1007/s00380-017-1054-8.

[234] E. Crosas-Molist *et al.*, "Vascular smooth muscle cell phenotypic changes in patients with marfan syndrome," *Arterioscler. Thromb. Vasc. Biol.*, vol. 35, no. 4, pp. 960–972, 2015, doi: 10.1161/ATVBAHA.114.304412.

[235] X. Shi *et al.*, "TGF-??/Smad3 stimulates stem cell/developmental gene expression and vascular smooth muscle cell de-differentiation," *PLoS One*, vol. 9, no. 4, 2014, doi: 10.1371/journal.pone.0093995.

[236] N. Mao, T. Gu, E. Shi, G. Zhang, L. Yu, and C. Wang, "Phenotypic switching of vascular smooth muscle cells in animal model of rat thoracic aortic aneurysm," *Interact. Cardiovasc. Thorac. Surg.*, vol. 21, no. 1, pp. 62–70, 2015, doi: 10.1093/icvts/ivv074.

[237] C. E. Gacchina and A. Ramamurthi, "Impact of pre-existing elastic matrix on TGFβ1 and HA oligomer-induced regenerative elastin repair by rat aortic smooth muscle cells," *J. Tissue Eng. Regen. Med.*, vol. 5, no. 2, pp. 85–96, Feb. 2011, doi: 10.1002/term.286.

[238] Y. Liu, B. Deng, Y. Zhao, S. Xie, and R. Nie, "Differentiated markers in undifferentiated cells: expression of smooth muscle contractile proteins in multipotent bone marrow mesenchymal stem cells.," *Dev. Growth Differ.*, vol. 55, no. 5, pp. 591–605, 2013, doi: 10.1111/dgd.12052.

[239] C. Rodríguez, J. Martínez-González, B. Raposo, J. F. Alcudia, A. Guadall, and L. Badimon, "Regulation of lysyl oxidase in vascular cells: Lysyl oxidase as a

new player in cardiovascular diseases," *Cardiovasc. Res.*, vol. 79, no. 1, pp. 7–13, 2008, doi: 10.1093/cvr/cvn102.

[240] C. Min *et al.*, "The tumor suppressor activity of the lysyl oxidase propeptide reverses the invasive phenotype of Her-2/neu-driven breast cancer," *Cancer Res.*, vol. 67, no. 3, pp. 1105–1112, 2007, doi: 10.1158/0008-5472.CAN-06-3867.

[241] B. Fogelgren *et al.*, "Cellular fibronectin binds to lysyl oxidase with high affinity and is critical for its proteolytic activation," *J. Biol. Chem.*, vol. 280, no. 26, pp. 24690–24697, 2005, doi: 10.1074/jbc.M412979200.

[242] Q. Xiao and G. Ge, "Lysyl oxidase, extracellular matrix remodeling and cancer metastasis," *Cancer Microenviron.*, vol. 5, no. 3, pp. 261–273, 2012, doi: 10.1007/s12307-012-0105-z.

[243] R. Kinsey *et al.*, "Fibrillin-1 microfibril deposition is dependent on fibronectin assembly," *J. Cell Sci.*, vol. 121, no. 16, pp. 2696–2704, 2008, doi: 10.1242/jcs.029819.

[244] D. F. Mosher, "Assembly of fibronectin into extracellular matrix," *Curr. Opin. Struct. Biol.*, vol. 3, no. 2, pp. 214–222, 1993, doi: 10.1016/S0959-440X(05)80155-1.

[245] J. E. Wagenseil and R. P. Mecham, "New insights into elastic fiber assembly," *Birth Defects Res. Part C - Embryo Today Rev.*, vol. 81, no. 4, pp. 229–240, 2007, doi: 10.1002/bdrc.20111.

[246] A. W. Clarke, S. G. Wise, S. A. Cain, C. M. Kielty, and A. S. Weiss,

"Coacervation is promoted by molecular interactions between the PF2 segment of fibrillin-1 and the domain 4 region of tropoelastin," *Biochemistry*, vol. 44, no. 30, pp. 10271–10281, 2005, doi: 10.1021/bi050530d.

[247] D. Lorena, I. A. Darby, D. P. Reinhardt, V. Sapin, J. Rosenbaum, and A. Desmoulière, "Fibrillin-1 expression in normal and fibrotic rat liver and in cultured hepatic fibroblastic cells: modulation by mechanical stress and role in cell adhesion.," *Lab. Invest.*, vol. 84, no. 2, pp. 203–212, 2004, doi: 10.1038/labinvest.3700023.

[248] M. Horiguchi *et al.*, "Fibulin-4 conducts proper elastogenesis via interaction with cross-linking enzyme lysyl oxidase," *Proc. Natl. Acad. Sci. U. S. A.*, vol. 106, no. 45, pp. 19029–19034, 2009, doi: 10.1073/pnas.0908268106.

[249] P. G. Drewes *et al.*, "Pelvic organ prolapse in fibulin-5 knockout mice: Pregnancy-induced changes in elastic fiber homeostasis in mouse vagina," *Am. J. Pathol.*, vol. 170, no. 2, pp. 578–589, 2007, doi: 10.2353/ajpath.2007.060662.

[250] G. M. Northington, "Fibulin-5: Two for the price of one maintaining pelvic support," *J. Clin. Invest.*, vol. 121, no. 5, pp. 1688–1691, 2011, doi: 10.1172/JCI57438.

[251] J. a Evans, "Diaphragmatic defects and limb deficiencies - taking sides.," *Am. J. Med. Genet. A*, vol. 143A, no. 18, pp. 2106–2112, 2007, doi: 10.1002/ajmg.a.

[252] R. Choudhury *et al.*, "Differential regulation of elastic fiber formation by fibulin-4 and -5," *J. Biol. Chem.*, vol. 284, no. 36, pp. 24553–24567, 2009, doi:

10.1074/jbc.M109.019364.

[253] M. Crowther, S. Goodall, J. L. Jones, P. R. Bell, and M. M. Thompson, "Increased matrix metalloproteinase 2 expression in vascular smooth muscle cells cultured from abdominal aortic aneurysms.," *J. Vasc. Surg.*, vol. 32, no. 3, pp. 575–83, 2000, doi: 10.1067/mva.2000.108010.

[254] E. S. Kim, Y. W. Sohn, and A. Moon, "TGF-β-induced transcriptional activation of MMP-2 is mediated by activating transcription factor (ATF)2 in human breast epithelial cells," *Cancer Lett.*, vol. 252, no. 1, pp. 147–156, 2007, doi: 10.1016/j.canlet.2006.12.016.

[255] G. Martufi and T. C. Gasser, "Turnover of fibrillar collagen in soft biological tissue with application to the expansion of abdominal aortic aneurysms," *J. R. Soc. Interface*, vol. 9, no. 77, pp. 3366–3377, Dec. 2012, doi: 10.1098/rsif.2012.0416.

[256] C. B. Saitow, S. G. Wise, A. S. Weiss, J. J. Castellot, and D. L. Kaplan, "Elastin biology and tissue engineering with adult cells," *Biomol. Concepts*, vol. 4, no. 2, pp. 173–85, Jan. 2013, doi: 10.1515/bmc-2012-0040.

[257] S. Dahal, T. Broekelman, R. P. Mecham, and A. Ramamurthi, "Maintaining Elastogenicity of Mesenchymal Stem Cell-Derived Smooth Muscle Cells in Two-Dimensional Culture," *Tissue Eng. - Part A*, vol. 24, no. 11–12, pp. 979–989, 2018, doi: 10.1089/ten.tea.2017.0237.

[258] D. Seliktar, R. A. Black, R. P. Vito, and R. M. Nerem, "Dynamic mechanical conditioning of collagen-gel blood vessel constructs induces remodeling in vitro," *Ann. Biomed. Eng.*, vol. 28, no. 4, pp. 351–362, 2000, doi:

10.1114/1.275.

[259] L. Venkataraman and A. Ramamurthi, "Induced Elastic Matrix Deposition Within Three-Dimensional Collagen Scaffolds," *Tissue Eng. Part A*, vol. 17, no. 21–22, pp. 2879–2889, 2011, doi: 10.1089/ten.tea.2010.0749.

[260] C. Labarca and K. Paigen, "A simple rapid and sensitive DNA assayt procedure," *Anal. Biochem.*, vol. 102, pp. 344–352, 1980.

[261] L. Venkataraman, C. A. Bashur, and A. Ramamurthi, "Impact of Cyclic Stretch on Induced Elastogenesis within Collagenous Conduits.," *Tissue Eng. Part A*, vol. 20, no. 9–10, pp. 1403–1415, 2014, doi: 10.1089/ten.TEA.2013.0294.

[262] M. Coliege, "Suppression of aortic elastic tissue autofluorescence for the detection of viral antigen," vol. 155, pp. 151–152, 1979.

[263] X. Shi *et al.*, "TGF-β/Smad3 stimulates stem cell/developmental gene expression and vascular smooth muscle cell de-differentiation," *PLoS One*, vol. 9, no. 4, p. e93995, 2014, doi: 10.1371/journal.pone.0093995.

[264] J. Van Den Akker, B. G. Tuna, A. Pistea, A. J. J. Sleutel, E. N. T. P. Bakker, and E. Van Bavel, "Vascular smooth muscle cells remodel collagen matrices by long-distance action and anisotropic interaction," *Med. Biol. Eng. Comput.*, vol. 50, no. 7, pp. 701–715, 2012, doi: 10.1007/s11517-012-0916-6.

[265] D. Seliktar, R. A. Black, R. P. Vito, and R. M. Nerem, "Dynamic mechanical conditioning of collagen-gel blood vessel constructs induces remodeling in vitro," *Ann. Biomed. Eng.*, vol. 28, no. 4, pp. 351–62, 2000, doi: 10.1114/1.275.

[266] H. R. Kim *et al.*, "Actin polymerization in differentiated vascular smooth muscle cells requires vasodilator-stimulated phosphoprotein," *Am. J. Physiol. - Cell Physiol.*, vol. 298, no. 3, pp. 559–571, 2010, doi: 10.1152/ajpcell.00431.2009.

[267] C. U. Schräder *et al.*, "Elastin is heterogeneously cross-linked," *J. Biol. Chem.*, vol. 293, no. 39, pp. 15107–15119, 2018, doi: 10.1074/jbc.RA118.004322.

[268] T. Ushiki, "Collagen fibers, reticular fibers and elastic fibers. A comprehensive understanding from a morphological viewpoint," *Arch. Histol. Cytol.*, vol. 65, no. 2, pp. 109–26, 2002, doi: 10.1679/aohc.65.109.

[269] S. Katsuda, Y. Okada, and I. Nakanishi, "Abnormal accumulation of elastin-associated microfibrils during elastolysis in the arterial wall," *Exp. Mol. Pathol.*, vol. 52, no. 1, pp. 13–24, 1990, doi: 10.1016/0014-4800(90)90054-H.

[270] W. Lin, L. Xu, S. Zwingenberger, E. Gibon, S. B. Goodman, and G. Li, "Mesenchymal stem cells homing to improve bone healing," *J. Orthop. Transl.*, vol. 9, pp. 19–27, 2017, doi: 10.1016/j.jot.2017.03.002.

[271] Y. Haraguchi, T. Shimizu, M. Yamato, and T. Okano, "Concise Review: Cell Therapy and Tissue Engineering for Cardiovascular Disease," *Stem Cells Transl. Med.*, vol. 1, no. 2, pp. 136–141, 2012, doi: 10.5966/sctm.2012-0030.

[272] D. Kumar and B. Chandra, "Regenerative Medicine : Recent Advances and Potential Applications," vol. 03, pp. 1–5, 2016.

[273] T. Doetschman, M. Shull, A. Kier, and J. D. Coffin, "Embryonic stem cell model systems for vascular morphogenesis and cardiac disorders.,"

Hypertension, vol. 22, no. 4, pp. 618–629, Oct. 1993, doi: 10.1161/01.HYP.22.4.618.

[274] D. L. Hutton, E. A. Logsdon, E. M. Moore, F. Mac Gabhann, J. M. Gimble, and W. L. Grayson, "Vascular Morphogenesis of Adipose-Derived Stem Cells is Mediated by Heterotypic Cell-Cell Interactions," *Tissue Eng. Part A*, vol. 18, no. 15–16, pp. 1729–1740, Apr. 2012, doi: 10.1089/ten.tea.2011.0599.

[275] P. T. Brown, A. M. Handorf, W. Bae Jeon, and W.-J. Li, "Stem Cell-based Tissue Engineering Approaches for Musculoskeletal Regeneration," *Curr. Pharm. Des.*, vol. 19, no. 19, pp. 3429–3445, 2013, doi: 10.2174/13816128113199990350.

[276] D. C. Colter, R. Class, C. M. DiGirolamo, and D. J. Prockop, "Rapid expansion of recycling stem cells in cultures of plastic-adherent cells from human bone marrow," *Proc. Natl. Acad. Sci. U. S. A.*, 2000, doi: 10.1073/pnas.97.7.3213.

[277] O. K. Lee, T. K. Kuo, W. M. Chen, K. Der Lee, S. L. Hsieh, and T. H. Chen, "Isolation of multipotent mesenchymal stem cells from umbilical cord blood," *Blood*, 2004, doi: 10.1182/blood-2003-05-1670.

[278] L. Fouillard *et al.*, "Infusion of allogeneic-related HLA mismatched mesenchymal stem cells for the treatment of incomplete engraftment following autologous haematopoietic stem cell transplantation [8]," *Leukemia*. 2007, doi: 10.1038/sj.leu.2404550.

[279] A. De Becker and I. Van Riet, "Homing and migration of mesenchymal stromal cells: How to improve the efficacy of cell therapy?," *World J. Stem Cells*, vol. 8, no. 3, pp. 73–87, 2016, doi: 10.4252/wjsc.v8.i3.73.

[280] Ma. Gnecchi, Z. Zhang, A. Ni, and V. J. Dzau, "Paracrine mechanisms in adult stem cell signaling and therapy," *Circ. Res.*, vol. 103, no. 11, pp. 1204–1219, 2008, doi: 10.1111/j.1743-6109.2008.01122.x.Endothelial.

[281] M. Gnecchi, P. Danieli, G. Malpasso, and M. C. Ciuffreda, "Paracrine Mechanisms of Mesenchymal Stem Cells in Tissue Repair.," *Methods Mol. Biol.*, vol. 1416, pp. 123–46, 2016, doi: 10.1007/978-1-4939-3584-0_7.

[282] M. Mirotsou, T. M. Jayawardena, J. Schmeckpeper, M. Gnecchi, and V. J. Dzau, "Paracrine mechanisms of stem cell reparative and regenerative actions in the heart," *Journal of Molecular and Cellular Cardiology*, vol. 50, no. 2. pp. 280–289, 2011, doi: 10.1016/j.yjmcc.2010.08.005.

[283] D. M. Choumerianou, H. Dimitriou, and M. Kalmanti, "Stem Cells: Promises Versus Limitations," *Tissue Eng. Part B Rev.*, vol. 14, no. 1, pp. 53–60, Mar. 2008, doi: 10.1089/teb.2007.0216.

[284] A. L. Ponte *et al.*, "The in vitro migration capacity of human bone marrow mesenchymal stem cells: comparison of chemokine and growth factor chemotactic activities.," *Stem Cells*, vol. 25, no. 7, pp. 1737–45, 2007, doi: 10.1634/stemcells.2007-0054.

[285] I. Petit *et al.*, "Atypical PKC-ζ regulates SDF-1–mediated migration and development of human CD34+ progenitor cells," *J. Clin. Invest.*, vol. 115, no. 1, pp. 168–176, Jan. 2005, doi: 10.1172/JCI21773.

[286] U. M. Fischer *et al.*, "Pulmonary passage is a major obstacle for intravenous stem cell delivery: the pulmonary first-pass effect.," *Stem Cells Dev.*, vol. 18, no. 5, pp. 683–692, 2009, doi: 10.1089/scd.2008.0253.

[287] B. Rüster *et al.*, "Mesenchymal stem cells display coordinated rolling and adhesion behavior on endothelial cells.," *Blood*, vol. 108, no. 12, pp. 3938–3944, Dec. 2006, doi: 10.1182/blood-2006-05-025098.

[288] J. Leibacher and R. Henschler, "Biodistribution, migration and homing of systemically applied mesenchymal stem/stromal cells," *Stem Cell Res. Ther.*, vol. 7, p. 7, Jan. 2016, doi: 10.1186/s13287-015-0271-2.

[289] A. Kurtz, "Mesenchymal stem cell delivery routes and fate," *Int. J. stem cells*, vol. 1, no. 1, pp. 1–7, Nov. 2008, doi: 10.15283/ijsc.2008.1.1.1.

[290] S. Koichi, M. R. N., and L. Peter, "Inflammation and Cellular Immune Responses in Abdominal Aortic Aneurysms," *Arterioscler. Thromb. Vasc. Biol.*, vol. 26, no. 5, pp. 987–994, May 2006, doi: 10.1161/01.ATV.0000214999.12921.4f.

[291] M. Liao *et al.*, "Plasma cytokine levels and risks of abdominal aortic aneurysms: A population-based prospective cohort study," *Ann. Med.*, vol. 47, no. 3, pp. 245–252, 2015, doi: 10.3109/07853890.2015.1019916.

[292] W. F. Johnston *et al.*, "Genetic and pharmacologic disruption of interleukin-1β signaling inhibits experimental aortic aneurysm formation," *Arterioscler. Thromb. Vasc. Biol.*, vol. 33, no. 2, pp. 294–304, 2013, doi: 10.1161/ATVBAHA.112.300432.

[293] M. Nishihara *et al.*, "The role of IL-6 in pathogenesis of abdominal aortic aneurysm in mice," *PLoS One*, vol. 12, no. 10, pp. e0185923–e0185923, Oct. 2017, doi: 10.1371/journal.pone.0185923.

[294] M. M. S. *et al.*, "Role of Interleukin 17 in Inflammation, Atherosclerosis, and Vascular Function in Apolipoprotein E–Deficient Mice," *Arterioscler. Thromb. Vasc. Biol.*, vol. 31, no. 7, pp. 1565–1572, Jul. 2011, doi: 10.1161/ATVBAHA.111.227629.

[295] W. Xiong, J. MacTaggart, R. Knispel, J. Worth, Y. Persidsky, and B. T. Baxter, "Blocking TNF-α Attenuates Aneurysm Formation in a Murine Model," *J. Immunol.*, vol. 183, no. 4, pp. 2741 LP – 2746, Aug. 2009, doi: 10.4049/jimmunol.0803164.

[296] D. Valerie *et al.*, "Matrix Metalloproteinase-2 Production and Its Binding to the Matrix Are Increased in Abdominal Aortic Aneurysms," *Arterioscler. Thromb. Vasc. Biol.*, vol. 18, no. 10, pp. 1625–1633, Oct. 1998, doi: 10.1161/01.ATV.18.10.1625.

[297] C. Tarín *et al.*, "Lipocalin-2 deficiency or blockade protects against aortic abdominal aneurysm development in mice," *Cardiovasc. Res.*, vol. 111, no. 3, pp. 262–273, May 2016, doi: 10.1093/cvr/cvw112.

[298] C. T. W.G., B. K. G., W. G. M.A., C. J. M., and S. Alberto, "Stromelysin-1 (Matrix Metalloproteinase-3) and Tissue Inhibitor of Metalloproteinase-3 Are Overexpressed in the Wall of Abdominal Aortic Aneurysms," *Circulation*, vol. 105, no. 4, pp. 477–482, Jan. 2002, doi: 10.1161/hc0402.102621.

www.ingramcontent.com/pod-product-compliance
Lightning Source LLC
LaVergne TN
LVHW040016200726
843493LV00005B/1287